100 GREATEST
MEDICAL
DISCOVERIES

ORLD

OOKS

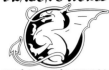

DRAGON'S WORLD

CHILDREN'S BOOKS

Dragon's World Ltd
Limpsfield
Surrey RH8 0DY
Great Britain

First published by Dragon's World 1995
Reprint 1995
© Dragon's World 1995

Text: Angela Royston
Editor: Kyla Barber
Copy Editor: Claire Watts
Designer: Mel Raymond
Design assistants: Karen Ferguson
                      Victoria Furbisher
Picture Research: Susan Trangmar
Art Director: John Strange
Editorial Director: Pippa Rubinstein

**The catalogue record for this book is
available from the British Library**

ISBN 1 85028 310 9

Printed in Italy

Contents

Introduction

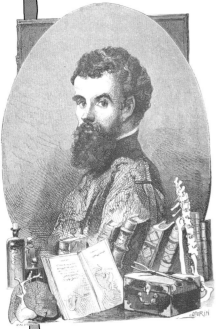

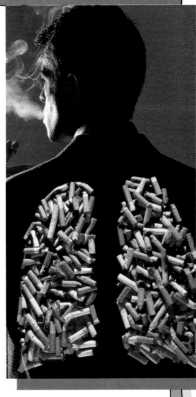

Have you been to the doctor or dentist recently? The experience was probably not too bad. If you need a filling, the dentist gives you an injection, and you don't feel any pain. If you have an ear infection, the doctor gives you an antibiotic and it feels better after a few days. Doctors now can prevent you getting a whole range of diseases. You may have already had chicken pox, but you have probably been vaccinated against mumps, measles, tetanus and polio. Yet when your great-grandparents were children, diseases like these killed many people.

In the nineteenth century, children were lucky just to survive to adulthood. Many babies died at birth and many more died of disease before they were five years old. Most families

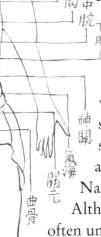

had ten, twelve, or more children, partly because parents did not know about contraception and partly because so many of their children died. Even simple operations, like removing tonsils or having a tooth taken out, were life-threatening. With no anaesthetic to ease the pain, can you imagine what it must have been like?

In medieval times, doctors even believed that the pus from an infected wound was a good thing. They thought that letting blood flow from the injured part of the body would help recovery. Even into the nineteenth century, doctors continued to take blood from patients to help them get better. One historian worked out that a single doctor in Paris shed more blood than all the fighting in the Napoleonic Wars! Although they did not often understand the causes of illness, doctors, from the earliest times, did their best to cure people. For hundreds of years ideas about illness were linked with religion and the forces of good and evil. It was thought that people fell ill because they had been wicked.

This book brings together one hundred advances in medicine and science that have improved the quality and length of our lives. Some advances, such as the discovery of penicillin, were made by lucky accidents, but most were the result of careful experiments, trial and error and the amazing dedication of doctors and scientists. But the war against disease is not yet won. Millions of people all over the world still do not have clean drinking water. Illnesses such as cancer and heart disease claim many lives in the developed parts of the world, and new diseases like AIDS cannot yet be cured. In years to come, scientists and doctors will cure these diseases too. Perhaps one day, you will make a medical discovery.

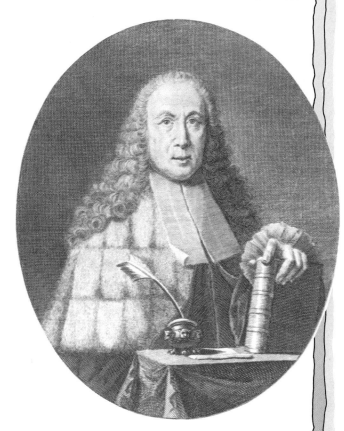

Andreas Vesalius (top left)
Giovanni Morgagni (above)
Acupuncture (bottom left)
Smoking as a major cause of death (top centre)
Closed chest cardiac massage (below)

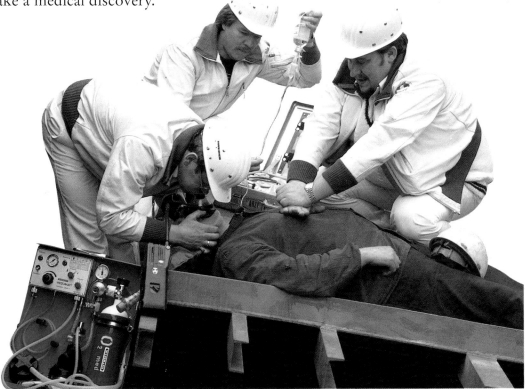

Trepanning

PREHISTORIC

Our prehistoric ancestors believed that boring a hole through the skull, an operation known as 'trepanning', would help to cure illness. For most of human history, people thought that pain and illness were caused by evil spirits. Witch doctors and shamans were employed to exorcize the spirits, but, if that failed, they might try trepanning.

Although we now know that trepanning is no cure for anything, it does show that even before people learned to write they were trying to find ways of curing illness. Trepanned skulls have been found all over the world, in France, Germany, North Africa, New Zealand and South America. It was particularly popular in Peru where skulls have been found with four and five holes in them. We know that some people even survived the operation because their skulls contain holes that have healed. Trepanning was carried out for thousands of years, well into the Middle Ages.

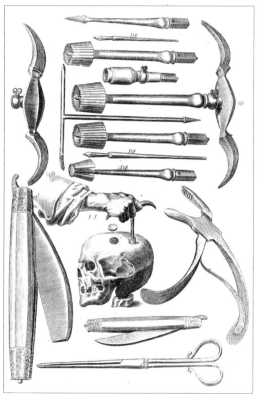

▲ Some of the instruments, used for trepanning, that you might have found in a surgeon's collection. The instruments are called trephines, and come in all shapes and sizes.

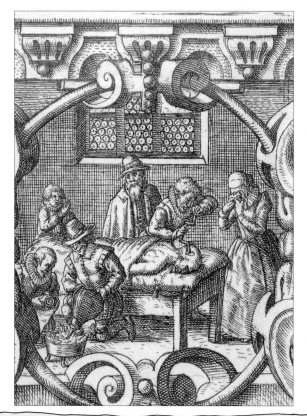

The instrument used for trepanning was rather like a carpenter's bit with a handle. If the patient lived, the wound in the head was covered with a piece of stone, shell, plant gourd or even with silver or gold.

◀ Trepanning operations were carried out before the invention of anaesthetics (the patient had to be held down) and were performed to treat headaches and to cure insanity.

Diagnosis

BABYLON 1000 BC

In about 450 BC, the Greek traveller Herodotus reported that in Babylon sick people were put on display so that people who passed by could say what they thought was wrong. But as long ago as 1000 BC, the Babylonians had a much better way of diagnosing illness. It was written on forty clay tablets and called *The Treatise of Medical Diagnosis and Prognosis*. It describes the symptoms of 3,000 different illnesses with their likely outcome, or 'prognosis'. Babylonians believed that illness was caused by evil spirits entering the body, but they observed the symptoms in great detail according to which part of the body was affected and noted how they changed during the day. Priests were employed to get rid of the spirits by chanting incantations and giving the patient medicines made from mustard, turpentine, pine and other herbs.

Babylonian doctors were the first to be regulated by law. The 'Hammurabi Code' laid down what a surgeon could charge for an operation which saved someone's life: ten shekels of silver for a lord, five for a commoner but only two for a slave. If the operation failed and the person died, the surgeon's hand was cut off.

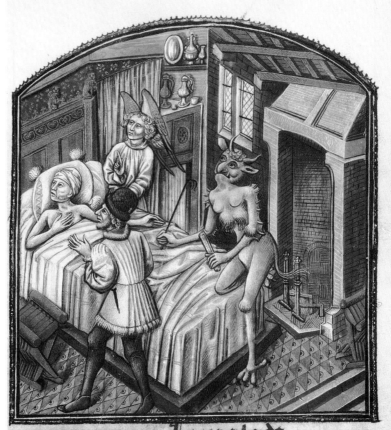

Le malade
uant le disciple entent
tel exemple / il prent a
souftraire son cuer et
t son entendement hors
de toutes choses mondaines. et ta

▶ The health of a person was thought to reflect the battle between good and bad, so part of a doctor's job was to drive away the forces of evil.

9

Operating to save sight

Susrata INDIA 750 BC

Cataract is most common among old people. The lens of the eye becomes cloudy and eventually blocks all light from entering the eye. If the lens is removed, the person can see light again, although they need glasses to see clearly. Even today this simple, but delicate, operation can seem like a miracle. Imagine the effect it must have had when Susrata first performed it in India nearly 3,000 years ago!

It was not the only operation Susrata carried out. In about 750 BC, he wrote a medical treatise called *Susruta Samhita* which deals exclusively with surgery. Surgeons in India carried out more operations than anywhere else in the ancient world. Indian doctors had a thorough training. They had to memorize *Susruta Samhita* before they were allowed to operate on people, and they practised their surgical skills by making incisions into pickles, cutting open leather bags filled with slime and burning or 'cauterizing' pieces of meat.

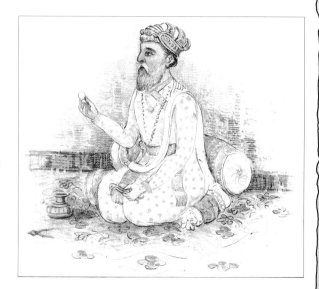

Indian doctors at the time of Susrata had 121 different steel instruments, including scalpels, probes and catheters. Instead of stitches, they used large ants to pinch the edges of a wound together until it healed. Once the pincers were gripping the flesh, they cut off the ants' bodies.

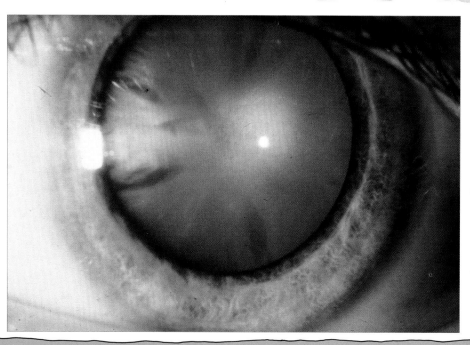

◄ The eye looks cloudy because this person is suffering from cataract. About one and a quarter million people in the world go blind due to cataracts each year.

Acupuncture

CHINA C. 450 BC

Recently some people in Europe and America have been amazed to find that acupuncture has helped them to give up smoking or allowed them to have painful operations without an anaesthetic. But acupuncture has been used in China for thousands of years. We know this from a book called *Nei Ching*, or the '*Manual of Physic*', written between 479 and 300 BC. It takes the form of a conversation set in about 2500 BC between Emperor Huangti and his prime minister and tells us much about Chinese medicine.

Instead of believing that evil spirits caused disease, the Chinese looked inside the body for the source of illness. They believe that everyone contains the opposing forces of yin and yang. Yin is dark, moist and female, while yang is bright, dry and masculine. Unless these forces are balanced, the body becomes ill. Acupuncture helps to restore the balance by allowing energy to enter or leave the body. Fine needles are inserted into the body at special acupuncture points.

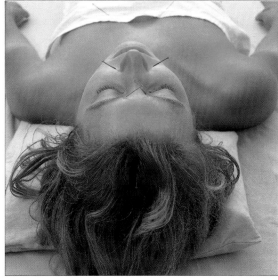

▲ This patient is using acupuncture to treat her hay fever. Chinese acupuncture is based on the theory that the surface of the body has close connections to the internal parts, so that by treating the surface, internal problems can be cured.

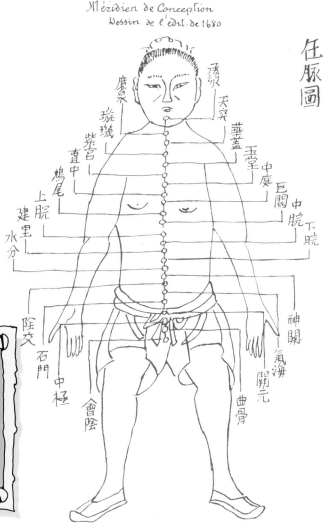

Mézidien de Conception
Dessin de l'édit. de 1680

▶ A Chinese diagram showing the 367 major acupuncture points on the body.

There are more than one hundred acupuncture points on each ear. Acupuncture points are along pathways that link to the organs but do not correspond to nerves. By sticking needles in points on the outer ear, pain and illness in other parts of the body may be relieved. (Do not try this yourselves – acupuncturists are experts.)

Caring for the patient

Hippocrates GREECE C. 400 BC

Just suppose you could not trust your doctor. Was he trying to poison you? Would she tell everyone your personal secrets? We know we can rely on our doctors to do their best for us because the standards laid down by Hippocrates over two thousand years ago are accepted throughout the world. Hippocrates is often known as 'the father of medicine'.

Hippocrates put the care of the patient before everything else. He overthrew the view that illness was caused by the gods and argued instead that it had natural causes, namely the four humours or fluids (see page 13), and should be treated scientifically. He realized that the environment can affect health and that the body can often heal itself.

He established a school and guild of medicine on the island of Cos in the Aegean Sea. He and his followers wrote a huge sixty-volume work called the *Hippocratic Collection* which includes many detailed case histories and describes how medicine should be practised.

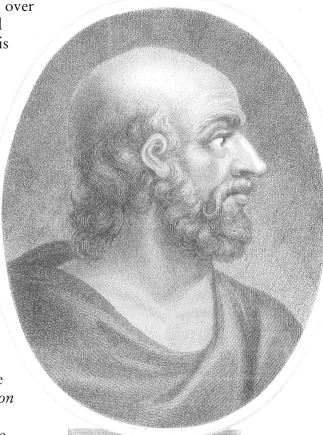

▼ The Greek physician, Hippocrates, wrote the first records of medical observations, and so created a new scientific base for medical practice.

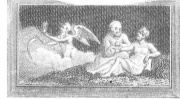

All the students at Hippocrates' school had to swear an oath. This is part of it: 'I swear ... that I will prescribe treatment to the best of my ability and judgement for the good of the sick, and never for a harmful or illegal purpose. I will give no poisonous drug.... Anything I see or hear should not be made public.'

Herbal remedies

Pedanius Dioscorides GREECE-ROME AD 45

Doctors in the ancient world may not have understood the causes of disease as we do today, but they knew that particular herbs could cure some of them. They mixed herbs together to make different medicines. Their skills were passed on and used by doctors for hundreds of years, thanks to the achievement of a pharmaco-botanist called Pedanius Dioscorides.

Pedanius Dioscorides was a doctor and a naturalist. He collected together all that was known about herbs and herbal remedies and wrote about them in *Materia Medica in Five Books*. He describes about 600 remedies of which about a fifth are still thought to be effective. Dioscorides was the undisputed authority on plant medicines for more than 1,500 years. His *Materia Medica* was translated into English in 1665 and is still in print.

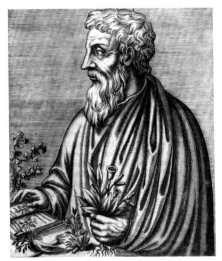

The Greeks believed that the body contains four fluids which corresponded to the four elements. Each fluid has its own characteristics and the balance of all four is vital for health.

Fluid	Element	Characteristic	Associated with
blood	air	hot & wet	blood
phlegm	water	cold & wet	brain
yellow bile	fire	hot & dry	liver
black bile	earth	cold & dry	spleen

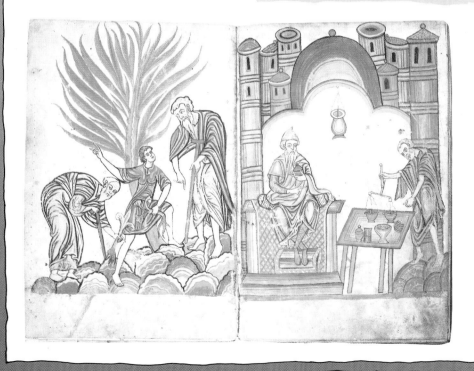

◀ A painting from a Latin manuscript showing the harvesting and preparation of herbal medicines. Many modern medicines are based on plant extracts.

Blood-letting and laudable pus

Galen of Pergamum GREECE-ROME AD 175

Galen was born in Pergamum in Turkey and studied medicine there and at Smyrna, Corinth and Alexandria. He became the doctor to a school of gladiators at Pergamum before settling in Rome where he was doctor to four emperors. He studied anatomy by cutting up pigs, monkeys and other animals. He thought that every organ must have a purpose and devised his own, usually incorrect, theories of how the body worked. He proved that veins and arteries carry blood not air, but thought that blood was made in the liver and taken, in the veins, to the organs where it was consumed.

Like Hippocrates, he believed in the four humours and thought that bleeding helped to restore the balance of the body's fluids. Patients were cut to allow the blood to flow. When wounds became infected and oozed pus, Galen thought that was good too. He called it 'laudable pus'.

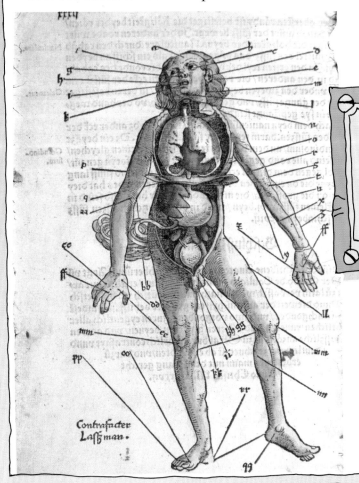

Galen pushed his ideas with bullying force. He quoted other people's theories only to destroy them with his own arguments. He produced such a complete system of medicine, linked to Christianity, that no one dared to challenge it for 1,500 years. Conflicting evidence was ignored because anyone who questioned Galen's theories risked being executed.

◀ The positions of the major blood-letting points on the body based on the teachings of Galen. Blood-letting, or 'breathing a vein' as it was known, was thought to help cure anything — from disease to over-eating!

14

Investigating brain injuries

Lanfranc of Milan FRANCE C. 1300

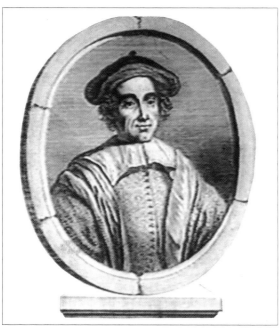

In the Middle Ages, doctors were educated at universities and their opinions were respected. Surgeons however, were often butchers or barbers who were untrained. Many were known as barber-surgeons and people only employed them as a last resort. Lanfranc, who was born in Milan but moved to France in 1290, said that surgery was equal to medicine and the two should not be separated.

Lanfranc was particularly interested in brain injuries and was the first to describe concussion. He used trepanning (see page 8) only when fragments were lodged in the skull or the membrane covering the brain was inflamed. To diagnose a fracture of the skull, he recommended that the surgeon or doctor tap the skull. If the noise rang clear, like an uncracked bell, there was no fracture. He later devised a better method. He tied a waxed string to one of the patient's teeth, pulled it taut and plucked it. The string gave different tones, depending on whether the skull was fractured!

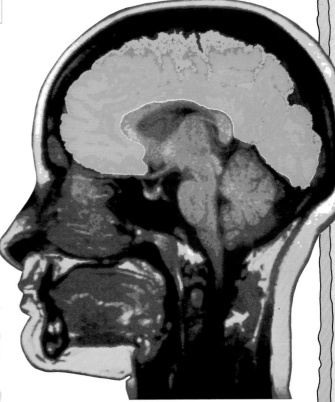

Concussion may occur when the brain is shaken, perhaps by a hit or fall on the head. The patient's vision and speech may be affected and they probably won't remember the accident. Anyone who has suffered concussion needs to be carefully watched to make sure there is no more serious injury.

▲ This computer-enhanced brain scan shows the major parts of a healthy brain. The technique uses radio waves to produce pictures of slices through the brain so that any problems can be picked up.

The science of anatomy

Andreas Vesalius BELGIUM 1543

Many of Galen's ideas about the human body (see page 14) were based on his dissections of animals. Cutting up a human body was illegal, and after Galen no one even studied the insides of animals. Doctors just accepted Galen's observations. It was not until the sixteenth century that people began to question his ideas.

Andreas Vesalius was professor in anatomy and surgery at Padua University. When he was a boy he cut open dead mice and birds to see what was inside. Later, at the University of Padua, he dissected human bodies. At first he ignored anything which did not agree with Galen, but he then realized that Galen had made mistakes. In 1543, he published *The Fabric of the Human Body*. It showed how nerves are connected to muscles, how bones are nourished and the complex structure of the brain. Immediately all other books became out of date and, by the end of the century, Vesalius' view of anatomy was generally accepted by doctors and surgeons.

Vesalius' assistants carried on his work. Gabriello Fallopio described the inside of the ear and the sex organs. Fallopian tubes which join the ovaries to the uterus are named after him. Bartolomuseo Eustachio gave his name to the Eustachian tubes which connect the ears to the throat.

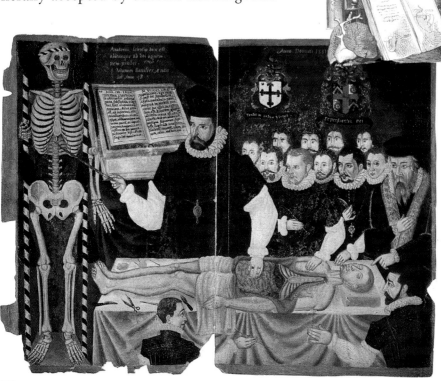

▲ Vesalius, the anatomist, became unpopular when he diagreed with the teachings of Galen, and was sentenced to death for dissecting human bodies. The sentence was reduced to a pilgrimage to Jerusalem, but he died on the return journey.

Dressings and ligatures

Ambroise Paré FRANCE 1545

Ambroise Paré was poorly educated yet he became a surgeon in the French army. He introduced many new surgical techniques and has been called the founder of modern surgery. When he started his career, boiling oil was poured onto wounds to stop them bleeding and becoming infected. The pain was so intense, many soldiers died. When oil ran out during the siege of Turin, Paré applied a dressing instead, with a mixture made from egg yolk, oil of roses and turpentine. It was not only less agonizing for the soldier, but the wound healed more quickly.

Many injuries led to amputation. A hot iron was often used to help stop the bleeding. But Paré developed a way of tying the arteries to stop them bleeding, called a 'ligature'. In 1545, he published *Method of Treating Wounds* which was translated and soon became the medical handbook for all of Europe's armies. Although his work was appreciated on the battlefield, it was laughed at by medical professors because Paré wrote in French instead of Latin – the traditional language of medicine.

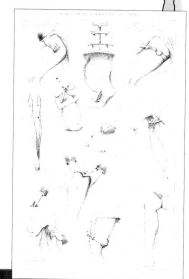

▶ Paré not only introduced many methods which could prevent soldiers from bleeding to death on the battlefield, but also developed the first, very basic, false limbs and teeth.

Ligatures are still used in operations today, although sometimes arteries are cauterized to seal them. The new technique, however, uses a laser beam and burns only the tiny area required.

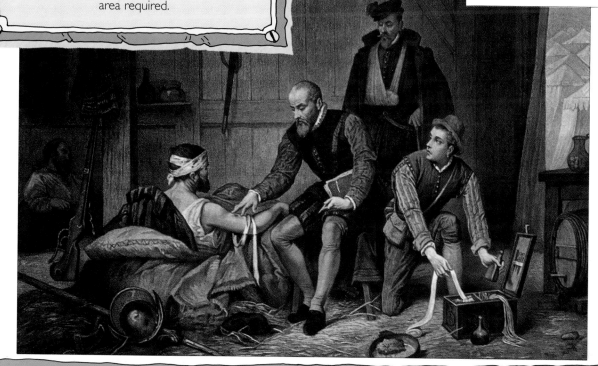

17

The science of embryology

Hieronymus Fabricius ITALY 1604

Hieronymus Fabricius extended the new zest for observing anatomy at first hand to the development of the unborn baby. People knew how babies were conceived, but what happened between conception and birth was more or less a mystery. Fabricius studied at Padua University and was taught anatomy by Gabriello Fallopio. After Fallopio died Fabricius took over as professor of anatomy and surgery in 1565. In 1600, he published *De formato foetu* (*On the formed foetus*) which describes the late stages of development of the foetus in different animals.

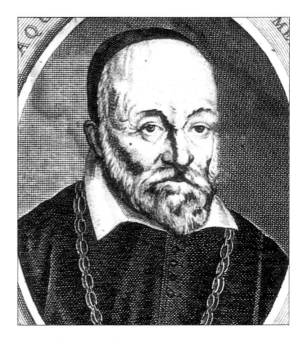

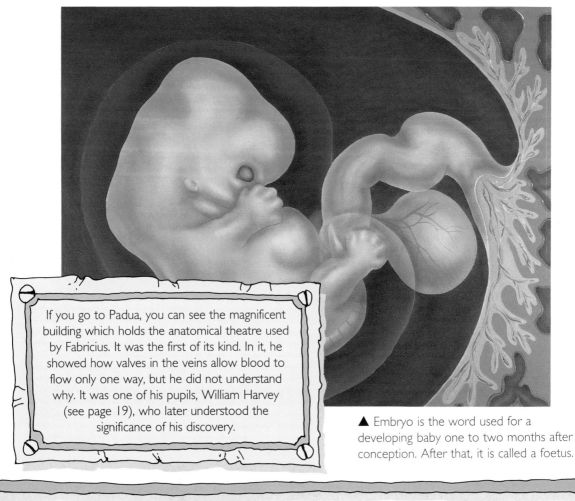

If you go to Padua, you can see the magnificent building which holds the anatomical theatre used by Fabricius. It was the first of its kind. In it, he showed how valves in the veins allow blood to flow only one way, but he did not understand why. It was one of his pupils, William Harvey (see page 19), who later understood the significance of his discovery.

▲ Embryo is the word used for a developing baby one to two months after conception. After that, it is called a foetus.

Blood circulation

William Harvey UNITED KINGDOM 1628

In 1603, William Harvey jotted in his notebook, 'The movement of blood occurs constantly in a circular manner and is the result of the beating of the heart'. This was a spectacular observation which totally contradicted Galen's view. Why did Harvey not publish it until twenty-five years later?

Because his theory contradicted Galen, Harvey had to be sure he was right. For years, he meticulously observed and experimented. He used a syringe to inject dye into the blood vessels of animals. Later, he dissected the animals to see where the blood had gone. He dissected the heart and studied its valves. By careful reasoning, he deduced that the heart pumped blood around the body. Even so when he eventually published his *Anatomical Treatise on the Movement of the Heart and Blood* in 1628, he was laughed at. Many doctors called him 'crack-brained' and said that his theory was absurd, impossible and harmful. Before he died in 1657, however, they had to agree that Harvey was right.

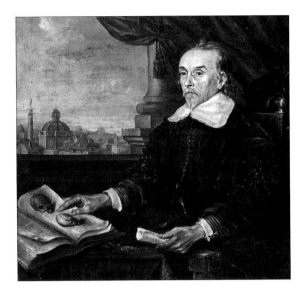

▼ Harvey's experiment shows that blood flows through the veins in only one direction. The normal flow in the vein is from the hand, back up the arm.

Harvey discovered that the heart consists of two pumps. Blood from the body goes from the veins into the right half of the heart and is pumped into the lungs where it collects oxygen. It then returns to the left half of the heart to be pumped through the arteries into the body. Valves inside the heart make sure that no blood flows back the wrong way.

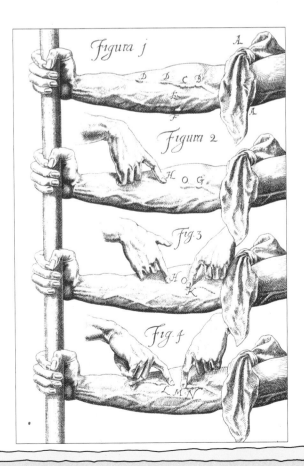

Obstetric forceps

Peter Chamberlain UNITED KINGDOM 1630

Today, the birth of a baby is usually a safe and happy event, but until recently many women and babies died in childbirth. Yet the invention which more than any other has made childbirth safer was kept secret for over a hundred years.

The Chamberlens were a family of male midwives. They fled to England from France in 1569 to escape religious persecution, and changed their name to Chamberlain. The success of their invention, the forceps, soon became known. They carried their instrument around in a wooden chest and went to great lengths to keep them secret. The woman in labour was blindfolded and everyone else was banished from the room. Listeners at the door heard strange noises. The Chamberlains banged sticks and rang bells to hide the clink of metal.

The Chamberlain family became rich but did not give away their secret until a few years before the last of them died in 1728. In 1733, Edmund Chapman published the first detailed description of forceps.

Babies are usually born head first. Forceps have two flat blades which curve slightly to fit round the baby's head. The blades are locked together and pulled gently but firmly. Once the head is free the rest of the body follows easily.

▼ In the foreground are two pairs of forceps originally used by Chamberlain and his family.

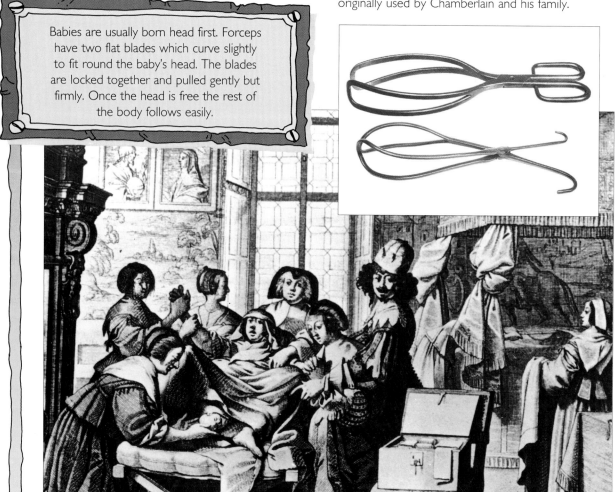

Bacteria

Anton van Leeuwenhoek

HOLLAND 1673

Anton van Leeuwenhoek was the first person to see bacteria and red blood cells under the microscope, yet he was neither a doctor nor a scientist. He was a draper who liked to make microscopes in his spare time. He made a new lens and microscope for each thing he observed. He studied fleas, aphids and ants and minute water creatures, which he called 'animalcules'. He made stronger lenses to look at blood, sperm and even bacteria. He wrote letters to the Royal Society describing his observations. In 1702, he wrote, 'Can there even now be people who still hold to the ancient belief that living creatures are generated out of corruption?' At that time most people believed that illness was generated from within the body. Proof of the connection between bacteria and disease, however, did not come until the end of the nineteenth century.

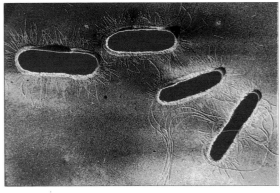

▲ These rod bacteria have been enlarged 4,000 times under a modern light microscope.

Leeuwenhoek was not the first person to realize the importance of bacteria. The Roman writer Varro thought that disease was probably caused by tiny animals that were too small to see. They were carried in the air and entered the body through the nose or mouth. In 1546, Girolamo Fracastoro wrote about 'disease-seeds' that were carried in the air.

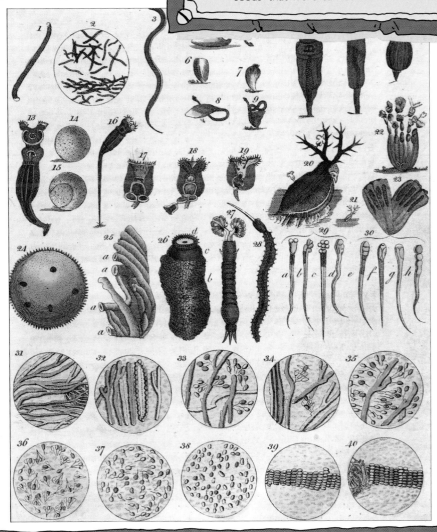

▶ Leeuwenhoek was able to see all sorts of microscopic creatures with his new light microscope.

Micro-organisms

G. Bonomo 1687

Although Leeuwenhoek had seen and described bacteria in 1673, most doctors continued to believe that illness was caused by bad air, hygiene and environment. Many who did accept that disease was caused by parasites still thought that they were generated inside the body. They pointed to the way maggots appeared 'from nowhere' in rotting meat. Even after Francesco Redi showed, in 1668, that no maggots appeared if you stopped flies getting to the meat, the theory still hung on.

Bonomo was the first person to link a particular parasite with the disease scabies, which makes the skin very itchy. Through a microscope he saw 'a minute living creature' which was shaped like a whitish tortoise with 'a little dark upon the back, with some thin, long hairs'. He saw that the animals moved freely onto anything the patient touched, particularly towels, sheets, gloves, handkerchiefs and clothes, and he realized they could pass on to anyone who touched those things too.

▲ The scabies parasite, as seen down a microscope. The female mite burrows into human skin and lays her eggs which cause itching and can cause infection.

Because of Bonomo's work, we know how important it is to wash your hands after going to the toilet and before eating. Germs on your fingers and hands can very easily get into your stomach and make you ill.

Caesarean section

Jean Ruleau FRANCE 1689

When a Caesarean section is performed, the pregnant mother's abdomen and uterus are cut and the baby is lifted out. Today, this operation is performed to save the mother and baby from a difficult and dangerous birth, but before the invention of anaesthesia (see page 35) and antiseptics (see page 46) the operation itself was very dangerous. It was usually performed after the mother had died, in order to save the baby.

Caesarean sections on live mothers were uncommon, but not unknown. In 1500, a Swiss butcher called Jacob Nufer is said to have operated on his own wife, and both mother and child survived, but there is no proof. A hundred years later, in 1610, Jeremiah Trautman operated on a mother in Wittenberg. The woman lived only twenty-five days but the baby lived for nine years. Then in 1689, Jean Ruleau performed a successful

Caesarean operation in which both mother and child survived. By the end of the eighteenth century, Caesarean sections were becoming more common, although only between a quarter and a half of them were successful.

How did Caesarean section get its name? It is unlikely that Julius Caesar was born by Caesarean section, because it is known that his mother survived. It is more likely that it is named after a law passed by Julius Caesar when he was emperor of Rome, that, if a pregnant woman died, her unborn baby should be buried separately.

▼ An engraving of a Caesarean birth from a dead mother. Today this operation is performed when a baby is the wrong way up in the uterus before birth.

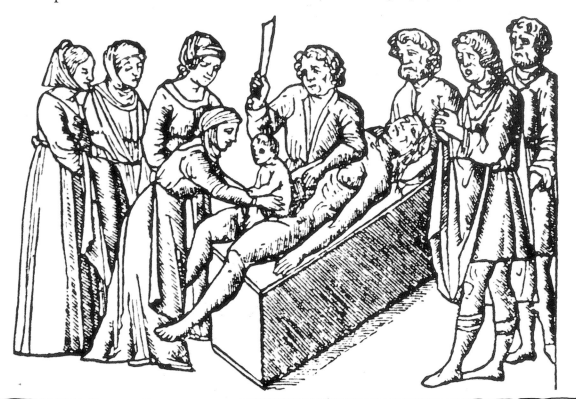

Pulse watch

John Floyer UNITED KINGDOM 1707

If you put your fingers between the veins and the edge of your wrist on the thumb side, you should be able to feel the regular beating of your pulse. As the heart beats, it produces a wave of pressure through the arteries, which can be felt at particular points in the body. Galen realized that taking a patient's pulse can give valuable information about health, but his judgements were not scientific.

John Floyer acknowledged Galen's skill in identifying various pulse beats, but he was appalled that even 1,500 years later, doctors were still not using any objective standard for measuring them. He said that the pulse should be counted using a watch or clock, and he had a special pulse watch made for timing sixty seconds. He published his findings in 1707 in a work called the *Physician's Pulse Watch*. But doctors largely ignored Floyer's advice for over a hundred years.

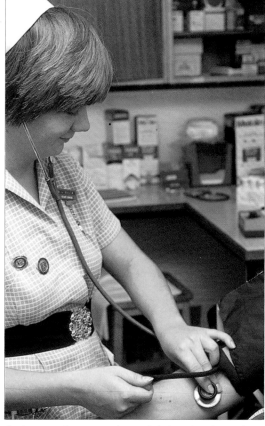

▲ A nurse listens to the patient's pulse through a stethoscope. The pulse rate depends upon level of activity, age and even size.

▶ Computer graphics showing the trace of a human pulse; heart beats.

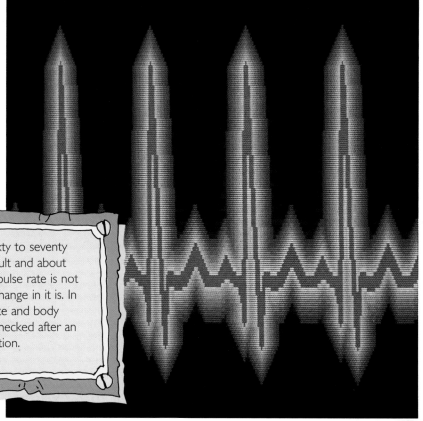

The normal pulse rate is sixty to seventy beats per minute for an adult and about eighty for a child. The actual pulse rate is not so important, but a sudden change in it is. In today's hospitals, pulse rate and body temperature are constantly checked after an accident or operation.

The prevention of scurvy

James Lind UNITED KINGDOM 1753

Sailors in the eighteenth century were used to drinking rum, but James Lind, a Scottish naval surgeon, introduced another drink on board ship – lemon juice. When Lind became a ship's surgeon in the Navy, many sailors suffered from scurvy, particularly on long voyages. It was called the 'plague of the sea' and caused bleeding gums, skin and joints. People already knew that to stay healthy they needed to eat a balanced amount of protein, fats, carbohydrates and mineral salts. Ships often carried animals on board to provide a supply of fresh food, but they did not take fruit and vegetables, which would rot on a long journey. Lind suspected that scurvy was due to the ships' limited diet, and he systematically went about finding a cure. He divided his crew, all suffering from scurvy, into small groups and gave each group a different dietary supplement for fourteen days. He found that the group eating oranges and lemons were much better after just six days. He published his results in 1754, but ships' captains were slow to follow his advice and scientists were slow to follow up his work on what were later to be called 'vitamins'.

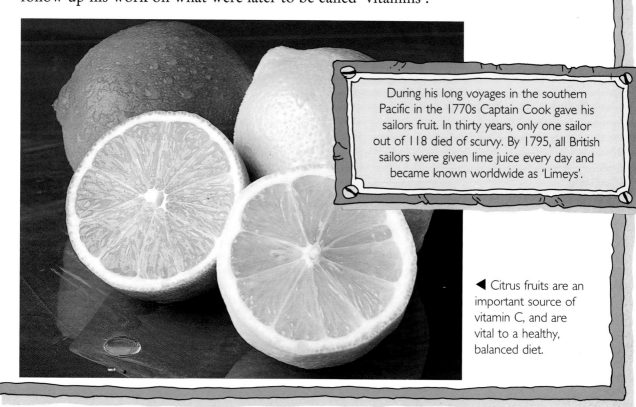

During his long voyages in the southern Pacific in the 1770s Captain Cook gave his sailors fruit. In thirty years, only one sailor out of 118 died of scurvy. By 1795, all British sailors were given lime juice every day and became known worldwide as 'Limeys'.

◀ Citrus fruits are an important source of vitamin C, and are vital to a healthy, balanced diet.

The science of pathology

Giovanni Battista Morgagni ITALY 1761

Cutting up dead bodies to find out the cause of death was not approved of in Greek and Roman times. The Christian Church did not allow it either until 1341. A few years later, the Black Death reached Europe. This plague killed over a third of the population of Europe, but even post-mortems could find no cure for it.

In 1712, Giovanni Battista Morgagni became professor of anatomy at Padua University. By then, thanks to Vesalius (see page 16) and others, anatomy had become an established subject and several doctors had published details of post-mortems. None, however, were as thorough or as comprehensive as the work Morgagni published in 1761. It was called *On the Seats and Causes of Disease* and it described over 500 post-mortems which compared diseased organs with healthy ones. He showed how the symptoms of a disease were linked to what had gone wrong inside the body. His work destroyed the theory of the four humours but doctors were slow to change their ideas.

Today, post-mortems are carried out whenever the cause of someone's death is uncertain. Police pathologists look for signs of murder, such as poison or suffocation.

▶ Two present-day pathologists are studying a slide made from a slice through a tumour. This special microscope allows them both to look at the same sample.

Respiration

Antoine Lavoisier France 1770–80

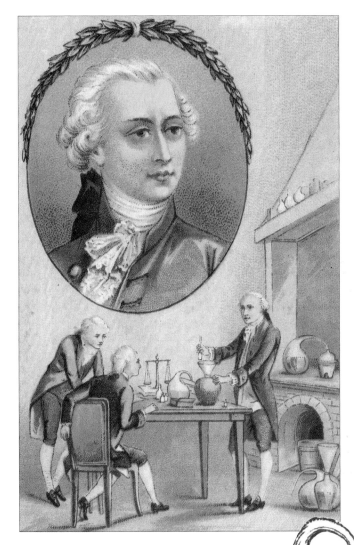

The British scientist Robert Boyle showed that a candle cannot burn without air and an animal in an airless space will die. He suggested that burning and breathing must somehow be similar. About a hundred years later, in 1774, the Swedish chemist, Carl Wilhelm Scheele, discovered oxygen, giving the French chemist Antoine Lavoisier the clue he needed to understand respiration.

By 1793, Lavoisier had shown how blood picks up oxygen in the lungs. He then described how the oxygen is burned inside the body to produce carbon dioxide and water. He used guinea pigs to measure the ratio between the amount of oxygen breathed in and the amount of carbon dioxide and water breathed out. He also showed that we breathe in more oxygen when we are active or eating than when we are relaxing.

Breathing and respiration are not the same. When you breathe, you take air into and out of your lungs. Once the air is in the lungs, the process of respiration takes over. Oxygen is taken up by the blood and used by the body.

▶ Lavoisier with the apparatus he used to investigate the properties of oxygen.

Smallpox vaccine

Edward Jenner UNITED KINGDOM 1798

After the plague, smallpox was the most widespread and feared disease in the world. It was well known that if someone recovered from an attack they would not catch it again. Jenner also knew that people who had suffered from cowpox, a much milder disease that milkmaids often caught, were also immune to smallpox.

Some doctors tried to inoculate people against smallpox by inserting pus from a smallpox sore into a scratch on their skin. It was called 'variolation' and was very risky. Sometimes it worked, but the patient always became ill and many died. Jenner decided to inoculate a small boy with pus from a cowpox sore instead. Six weeks later, he inoculated him with smallpox and the boy stayed healthy. Jenner inoculated twenty-three other people with cowpox before publishing his findings in 1798. Three years later, 100,000 people in Britain had been inoculated and by 1975 smallpox was wiped out from the whole world.

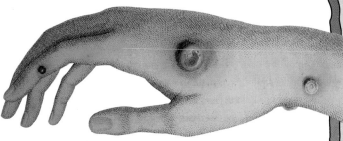

▲ A hand with cowpox sores. It was from sores like these that Edward Jenner was able to make his first vaccine

In 1803, a ship set sail for South America with twenty-two children on board. Two of them were vaccinated with Jenner's cowpox vaccine. Every ten days, two more were vaccinated from the arms of the previous pair. When the ship docked in Venezuela, the cowpox vaccine was still alive and ready to inoculate more people.

▼ Jenner performing his first vaccination. It took a whole year before this vaccine was considered safe.

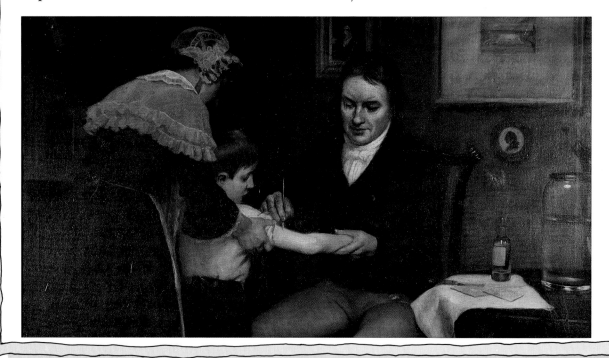

Homeopathy
Samuel Hahnemann GERMANY 1810

When Samuel Hahnemann trained as a doctor, blood-letting, forced vomiting and vile-tasting concoctions were believed to be the only remedies for most kinds of illnesses. Hahnemann found these remedies so unpleasant and useless, he stopped practising medicine. Thirty years later, he had founded a new system of medicine which was called 'homeopathy'.

When Hahnemann read that quinine was effective in treating malaria, he decided to try some on himself. He tested many substances, noted their effects and discovered that large doses of drugs that produce an illness in a healthy person will cure that illness in a sick person if given in very small doses. Hence the theory that 'like cures like'. In 1811, he published his findings.

In 1812, Paris was suffering from an epidemic of typhoid brought there from Moscow by Napoleon's defeated army. When people found that Hahnemann's medicines worked, they flocked to his door.

Homeoopathic Medicines

▲ A window displaying a variety of homeopathic medicines that are on sale today.

Homeopathy is still regarded as an 'alternative' medicine. A few illnesses seem to respond better to homeopathic remedies, but most are more effectively treated by conventional therapies. A homeopathic doctor tries to help the body restore its own natural balance.

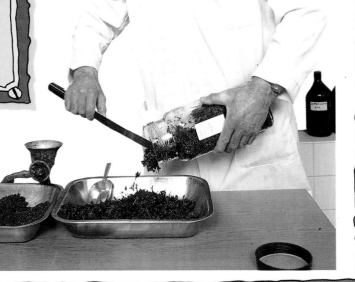

▶ Homeopathic medicines being made in the laboratory. Forty per cent of all modern medicines are made from plants.

The nervous system

Charles Bell UNITED KINGDOM 1811

Charles Sherrington UNITED KINGDOM 1891

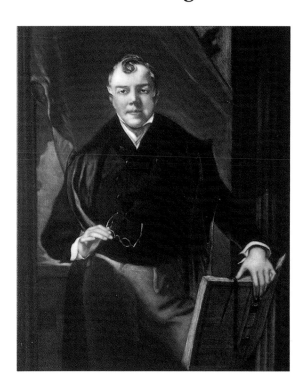

Building on the work other scientists had already carried out on the nervous system, Charles Bell found that there are two kinds of nerves, motor and sensory. Motor nerves control the muscles and sensory nerves take messages from the sense organs to the brain. Although we feel pain and other sensations in different parts of our body, we would not experience them without our brain. For example, light passes through our eyes, but we 'see' an image when our brain pieces together all the information.

Nearly fifty years after Charles Bell died, Charles Sherrington started work on spinal reflexes. Marshall Hall had already shown that: reactions to pain, blinking, coughing, and other automatic responses, link through the spine rather than the brain. Sherrington began a long series of experiments to find out which nerves in the spine did what. By removing the 'thinking' part of the brain from several animals he found out how the remaining spinal nerves acted together.

Sherrington knew that nerve messages are sent in the form of electrical impulses. He wondered how they crossed the 'gap' between one nerve and the next. Otto Loewi found the answer when he discovered that a chemical called 'acetyl choline', made in the body, carries the nerve messages.

◀ The brain is the controlling and coordinating centre of the nervous system.

The stethoscope

René Théophile Hyacinthe Laënnec FRANCE 1816

In ancient Greece, a doctor would always listen to a patient's heart by putting his ear to their chest, but the technique was forgotten until the Renaissance, when it became regular practice again. Then in 1816, a plump young woman came to Dr Laënnec complaining of heart trouble.

Laënnec was too embarrassed to put his ear to the woman's large bosom. He remembered seeing a child tap one end of a log while his friend listened at the other end. Laënnec seized a bundle of papers and rolled them into a tube. He put one end on the woman's chest and listened at the other end. To his amazement he heard the heart beating more clearly than he ever had before.

Laënnec made the first permanent stethoscope from a tube of wood twenty-three centimetres (nine inches) long and four centimetres (one and a half inches) wide. He described all the chest sounds he heard in his patients and linked many of them to different diseases.

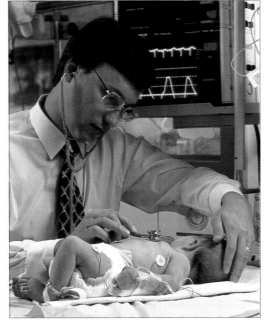

▲ A doctor uses a modern stethoscope to listen to a premature baby's heart. The word stethoscope means 'I look into the chest'.

Wooden stethoscopes were used until 1850 when they were replaced by rubber tubing. In 1852, an American doctor, George Cammann, added two earpieces. By 1878, microphones had been invented and one was connected to the chest piece to magnify the sound.

▼ Using one of the early stethoscopes was awkward and relied upon listening with only one ear.

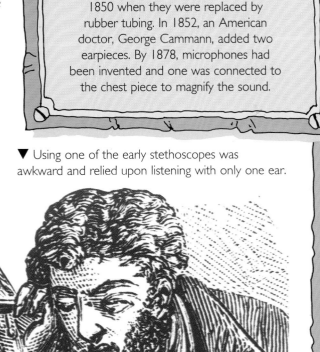

Blood transfusions

James Blundell UNITED KINGDOM 1829

The first successful blood transfusion was carried out in about 1665, when John Wilkins used a quill and a bladder to take blood from one dog and insert it into the vein of another dog. Two years later, the French doctor Jean Denis carried out the first medical transfusion when he inserted lamb's blood into the vein of a 15-year-old boy. The boy survived, but transfusions were so risky that few were attempted until the nineteenth century, when John Leacock became interested in them as a treatment for excessive bleeding. He concluded that it was safer to transfuse blood only between two animals of the same species.

James Blundell followed Leacock's advice. He began using a syringe to transfuse blood from his assistants to patients he knew were already dying. In 1829, he successfully gave blood from one of his assistants to a woman who was haemorrhaging after childbirth. The woman survived. As more transfusions were attempted, however, problems emerged. Sometimes the new blood mixed in successfully, but at other times it clumped together. These problems were later solved by Karl Landsteiner (see page 63) who studied blood groups.

Today over two million blood transfusions are carried out in the United States every year. Adults have about six litres (eight and a half pints) of blood. It is possible to lose up to a quarter of your blood and still survive, but any greater loss than that would certainly need a blood transfusion.

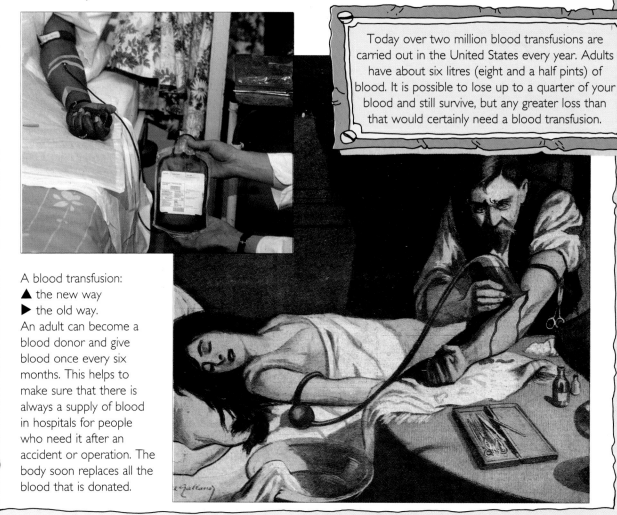

A blood transfusion:
▲ the new way
▶ the old way.
An adult can become a blood donor and give blood once every six months. This helps to make sure that there is always a supply of blood in hospitals for people who need it after an accident or operation. The body soon replaces all the blood that is donated.

The contraceptive diaphragm

Frederick Adolphe Wilde GERMANY 1838

Contraceptives are designed to allow couples to have sex without the woman becoming pregnant. As long ago as 3000 BC, women in Egypt were putting honey and crocodile dung inside their vaginas to try to prevent pregnancy. At that time, the best contraceptive was probably breast-feeding. When a woman is breast-feeding a baby, she is less likely to ovulate (or release an egg) which can then by fertilized by male sperm.

No one knows who invented the first male condom, but Japanese men are said to have worn sheaths of leather in the past, and European men sheep gut. In the sixteenth century, Gabriel Fallopio (see page 16) invented condoms of damp linen which continued to be used for the next 400 years, but more as protection from disease than as a contraceptive.

In 1838, Wilde invented a rubber diaphragm for women which could be fitted into the vagina to block off the neck of the womb. But in the nineteenth century, few women knew about contraceptives. Condoms were associated with prostitutes, and contraceptives of any kind were secret and illegal in many places.

▲ We now have sex education lessons at school.

▶ Margaret Sanger campaigned for birth control so that women could limit the size of their families.

The term 'birth control' was first used by the American Margaret Sanger. In 1914, she wrote a book called *Family Limitation* which encouraged people to use contraceptives. At the same time, Marie Stopes in the United Kingdom wrote books encouraging contraception.

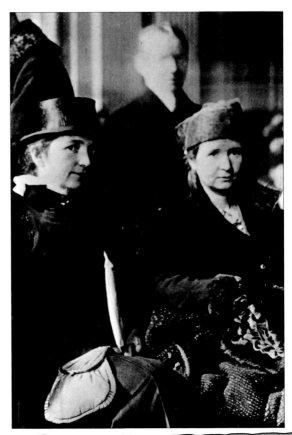

Public health

Edwin Chadwick UNITED KINGDOM 1842

William Gorgas PANAMA 1904

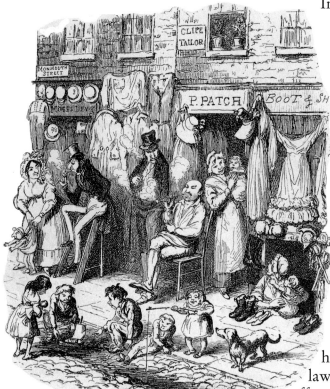

Parliament asked Chadwick to make his sanitary report because the smell of sewage in the nearby River Thames was making life unbearable in the House of Commons.

In the 1830s and 40s, people crowded into the growing cities of Britain, looking for work in the new factories. Charles Dickens' books describe the terrible conditions in which many people lived at the time. A civil servant, Edwin Chadwick, was asked to look into these conditions. He found that people who were poor were more likely to catch infectious diseases, and that they and their children were more likely to die. Only one eighth of Britain's towns had clean water. Chadwick's report said that rubbish should be removed from the streets and that water should be cleaned. He was unable, however, to get Parliament to pass laws strong enough to have much effect. His idea that disease is related to the environment did spread however, and public health slowly improved.

Sixty years later, on the other side of the Atlantic, another civil servant, William Gorgas, made an enormous improvement in public health by tackling the cause of yellow fever (see page 62). He had heard that this disease was caused by mosquitoes. He went to great lengths to destroy any possible breeding ground the mosquitoes might use and succeeded in ridding Panama of yellow fever.

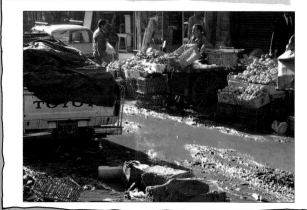

◄ A burst sewer floods this street in Cairo, Egypt. Even now, in poor countries, many lives are lost because of unhealthy living conditions.

General anaesthetic

William Morton USA 1846

Before the seventeenth century, patients who had to have an operation were given either alcohol, opium, henbane or mandrake root to dull the pain. However, the doses needed to knock them out were so large they were often fatal. After the seventeenth century, the patient was often simply held down during an operation and left to scream.

Anaesthetics were discovered almost by accident. In 1799, Humphry Davy discovered that if he breathed in nitrous oxide it made him laugh. Davy invited his friends to 'laughing gas' parties. Then, in 1815, Michael Faraday, another famous scientist, discovered that ether had a similar effect and invited his friends to enjoy it. It was not until the 1840s that the chemist C. T. Jackson suggested to one of his pupils, a dentist, that ether could be used as a local

The use of anaesthetics was quickly adopted and operations at last became less painful. However the Church objected to painkillers being used in childbirth. They argued that the Bible said that labour should be painful. In 1853, Queen Victoria used anaesthetic during childbirth, and it gradually became more widely accepted.

anaesthetic. When William Morton applied ether to a tooth he was about to drill, he noticed that the patient's whole mouth became numb. He wondered whether ether could be used as a general anaesthetic and experimented, first on animals then on himself. In October 1848, he arranged a public demonstration during which he painlessly removed a tumour from a patient's neck using ether as an anaesthetic. After that the use of ether spread quickly.

▼ Morton gives the patient ether during one of the earliest operations using general anaesthetic.

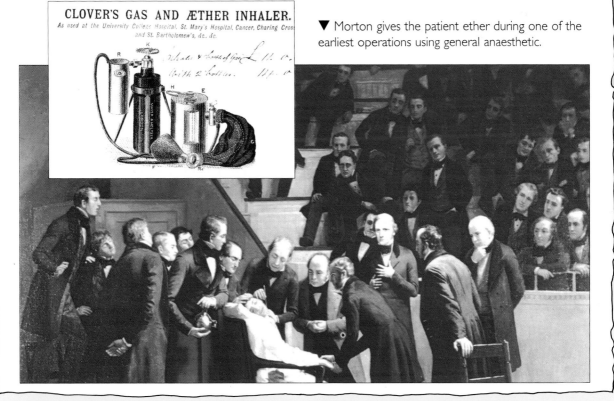

CLOVER'S GAS AND ÆTHER INHALER.
As used at the University College Hospital, St. Mary's Hospital, Cancer, Charing Cross and St. Bartholomew's, &c. &c.

The science of epidemiology

Peter Panum UNITED KINGDOM 1846

Infectious diseases, from the plague to a flu epidemic, can quickly spread through a group of people and even across a country or continent. Epidemiologists study how a disease spreads and what makes it die out, only perhaps to return again several years later. Peter Panum was one of the first to study epidemics in this way.

Today, measles is a mild childhood disease, but in Panum's day it was much more serious and killed thousands of people. In 1846, measles swept through the 7,864 people who lived in the Faroe Islands. Over 6,000 became ill and 102 died. The Danish government asked Panum to go to the Faroes to study the epidemic. Panum realized that populations isolated from a disease were more affected by it when it did strike. A devastating example occurred thirty years later when a British cruiser arrived in Fiji with someone suffering from measles on board. Within three months, a quarter of Fiji's population had died.

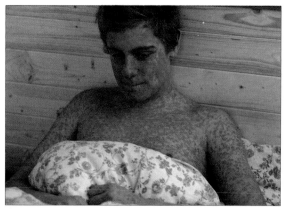

▲ This boy is suffering from measles.

Today most children in Europe, North America and Australasia are vaccinated against measles. The vaccine was not developed until 1963 but in just three years the number of cases in the United States had fallen from 482,000 to just 22,000.

▼ Conditions like these, in Indonesia, where there is overcrowding and dirty water flows through the streets, encourage the spread of infectious diseases.

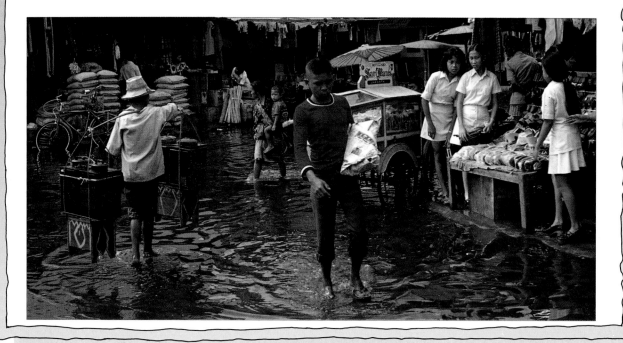

Infection theory

Ignaz Semmelweis HUNGARY 1847

Many mothers in the past survived childbirth only to die of childbed fever. They developed a high temperature and pain in the lower abdomen and died from heart failure. The disease most affected mothers who had given birth in hospital.

Most doctors thought that childbed fever was caused by 'miasma' or infectious air, but Ignaz Semmelweis noticed that a ward run by midwives was much less affected than a ward attended by medical students. The students came straight from dissecting rooms without washing their hands. Semmelweis thought that things which he called 'putrid particles' were being transferred from the bodies in the dissecting rooms to the mothers.

When Semmelweis ordered that all the students wash their hands with lime chloride, they protested strongly, but the number of deaths from childbed fever dropped dramatically. Semmelweis wrote a book about childbed fever, but people did not accept his theories about infection until after his death, when Joseph Lister (see page 46) publicly agreed with his ideas.

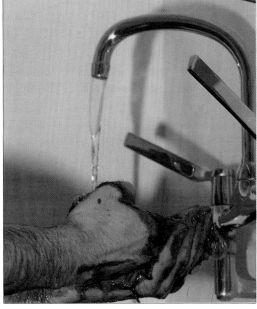

▲ A modern surgeon 'scrubbing up' before an operation. The cleaning solution looks orange in colour because it has an iodine base.

In 1865, Semmelweis was killed by the same bacteria that cause childbed fever. He cut his hand and contracted blood poisoning. He was taken into hospital but died shortly afterwards.

▼ A ward in the New Hospital for Women, where many women died after childbirth from childbed fever. The death rate for mothers fell greatly after hand-washing was made compulsory for all doctors.

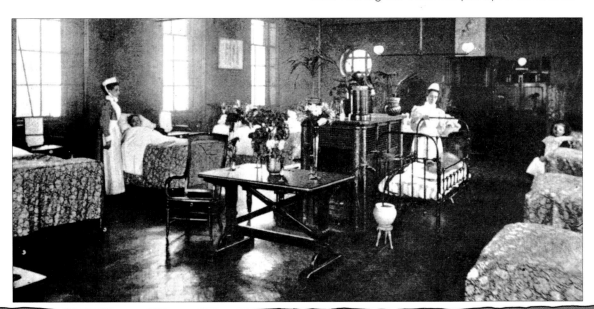

The ophthalmoscope
Hermann Ludwig von Helmholtz GERMANY 1851

If you have your eyes tested, the optician may use an ophthalmoscope to examine the inside of your eye by looking through the pupil, which is the black hole in the middle of the eye. This instrument was invented by the German scientist Hermann von Helmholtz in 1851. Before that date, doctors could only use a magnifying glass to examine the eye. With this new ophthalmoscope, they could see the blood vessels of the retina, at the back of the eyeball, and the optic nerve itself (which sends messages between the eye and the brain). This is the only place in the body that vessels and nerves can be looked at without cutting open the body. Doctors today use ophthalmoscopes to detect diseases like high blood pressure and diabetes.

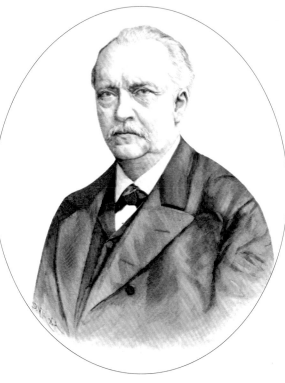

Nerve endings in the retina are sensitive to different colours of light. Some people have no endings sensitive to red, so they cannot tell red from green. We say that these people suffer from colour blindness.

▼ The doctor looks through an ophthalmoscope, which directs a fine beam of light into the eye and contains a magnifying glass which allows him to see the spot where the beam falls.

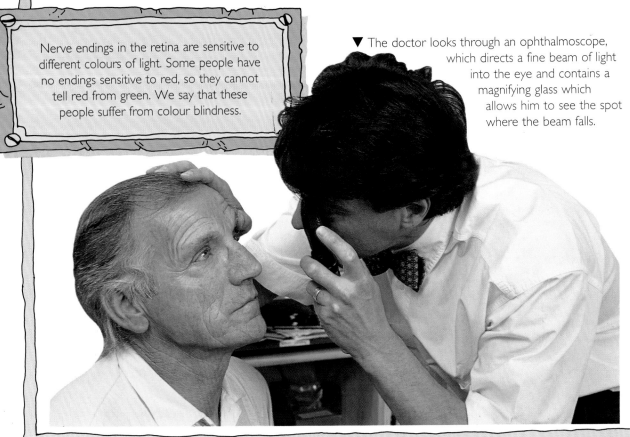

The hypodermic syringe

Charles Gabriel Pravaz FRANCE 1853

More than 1,500 years before Pravaz was born, Galen (see page 14) had used a syringe to inject blood vessels in the brain. More recently, Harvey (see page 19) used a hollow tube with a point at one end and a plunger inside, to inject dye into the blood to help him study its circulation. In 1713, a French surgeon, Dominique Anel, made a small syringe which ended in a very fine tube. He used it to operate on the tear duct in the eye.

All these syringes, however, could only be inserted into the body through natural body openings or by cutting into the skin first. When Pravaz added a fine, hollow needle to the end instead of the tube, he at last had a syringe which could inject directly under the skin. It was used two years later, in 1855, by a Scottish doctor, Alexander Wood, to inject a patient with morphia, a powerful painkiller. This was one of the earliest, successful forms of painkiller.

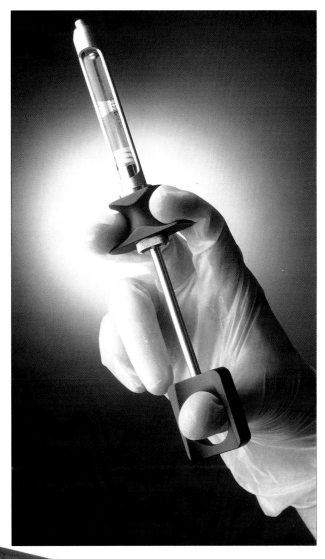

Hypodermic needles and syringes are used regularly in medicine today, to give injections of vaccines and drugs. Drugs injected straight into the blood act more quickly than those which have to be swallowed and digested first.

▲ Hypodermic syringes come in all shapes and sizes, depending on what they are used for. Some are used to remove a small sample of blood from a person for testing. Others are used to inject vaccines or anaesthetics.

Preventing cholera

John Snow UNITED KINGDOM 1854

Cholera is a disease which causes sudden, violent diarrhoea so that the patient loses large amounts of water and dies very quickly. One epidemic, which started in India in 1817, spread as far as London where it killed 7,000 people. In 1848, another epidemic arrived which killed 7,000 people in just one month. Most doctors thought that cholera was spread as a 'badness' in the air, but Dr Snow disagreed. He wrote a pamphlet saying that since cholera only affected the digestive system the infection must be swallowed. He suggested that drinking water that had been poisoned by infected sewage could be a cause.

No one listened to Snow, however, until cholera struck again in 1853 and 700 people died in one small area of Soho in London. Snow suspected a local water pump and persuaded the officials to take away the pump's handle. The epidemic ended a few days later. It took many months of research, interviewing survivors of the disease, before it was proved that the water in the pump had indeed been contaminated with cholera.

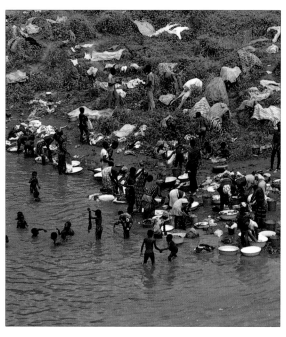

▲ Here, on the Ivory Coast, there is no clean water so people have to use river water for everything.

◄ One of the earliest filtered water pumps. This one provided clean water for the city of Paris.

Cholera is still found where people live in overcrowded and poor conditions. However it is not the overcrowding that causes the disease, but infected drinking water. Even after Snow's theory was proved, it was ignored, until 1883, many years after Snow's death, when Robert Koch identified the microbe responsible.

Understanding digestion

Claude Bernard FRANCE 1857

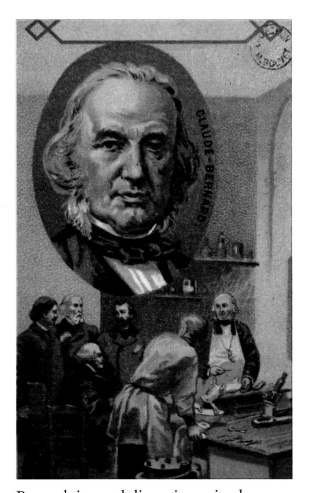

sugar in it a day later. In 1857, he isolated a substance which he called 'glycogen' and later showed that it changed to sugar in the liver. He also showed that the pancreas was involved in digesting fat, not in producing saliva as was previously supposed.

Digestion is a complicated process in which molecules of food are broken down into simpler units. Milk, for example, is broken down into fatty acid, sugar, proteins and vitamins. The substances the body needs are absorbed into the blood, the rest pass on through the gut and out of the anus.

By studying and dissecting animals, Claude Bernard discovered much about the way animals and humans digest food. He carried out his research with painstaking care. He was determined that every medical theory he had would be drawn from experiments. Any questions they raised would be answered only by more experiments. There was no room, he said, for speculation. Only his wife had doubts about the way he worked. She was a member of a society opposed to cruelty to animals.

Bernard's methods, however, were very successful. Although he had fed one animal on a sugar-free diet, he found sugar in its liver. After washing all the sugar out of the liver he again found

▼ The human digestive system. Food passes from the mouth, down to the stomach, through the small intestine and colon (large intestine) to the rectum and out through the anus. Chemicals in your body act on the food and help to break it down so that it can be used for energy and growth.

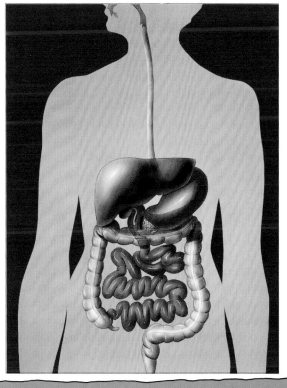

Germ theory

Louis Pasteur FRANCE 1857

Louis Pasteur was a scientist rather than a doctor, yet, by luck, his discoveries were to be of enormous value to medicine. In 1854, he was asked to study the problems of the wine and beer industries in Lille. As the alcohol fermented it sometimes went sour. In 1857, Pasteur announced that the fermentation was caused by micro-organisms in the yeast, not by a chemical reaction as had previously been supposed. He also discovered that micro-organisms turned milk sour. When he proved that these micro-organisms were carried in the air and were not 'spontaneously generated',

Pasteur realized that he had found the cause not only of fermentation and rotting, but of disease too. Milk also carried the micro-organisms of tuberculosis and typhoid. He discovered that if the milk was heated to a certain temperature for a certain time, the micro-organisms were all killed. The process is known as 'pasteurization' and is still used to make milk safe and to treat food before it is canned.

▼ Louis Pasteur in his laboratory where he developed the process of pasteurization. He found that bacteria are destroyed when they are heated to 62°C for thirty minutes, or by 'flash' heating to higher temperatures for less than one minute.

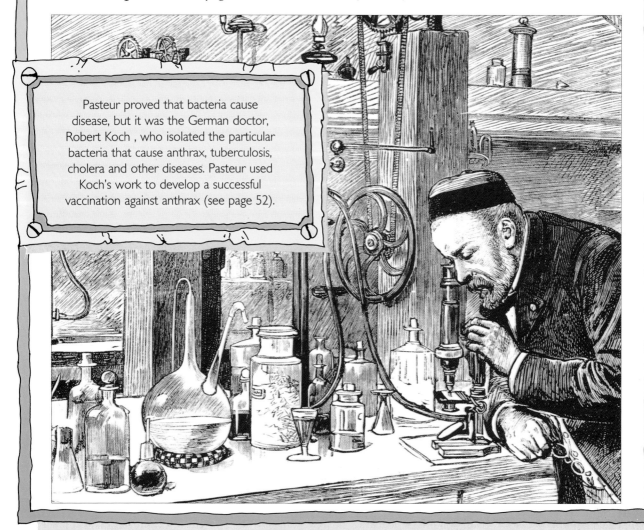

Pasteur proved that bacteria cause disease, but it was the German doctor, Robert Koch , who isolated the particular bacteria that cause anthrax, tuberculosis, cholera and other diseases. Pasteur used Koch's work to develop a successful vaccination against anthrax (see page 52).

Cellular division

Rudolf Virchow GERMANY 1858

In 1839, German anatomist Theodor Schwann had discovered that animals as well as plants are made of cells. He concluded that cells are the basic units of life but he thought they arose spontaneously from a formless substance which he called 'blastema'. Rudolf Virchow proved he was wrong.

In 1858, Virchow published an article in which he said that every cell comes from another cell. Life begins when a fertilized egg cell divides and divides again into the billions of cells which make up a human. He also believed that all diseases come from abnormal changes in cells. He correctly identified the abnormal cell in leukaemia, but he was reluctant to admit that many diseases were actually caused by bacteria.

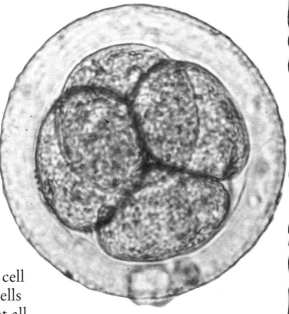

▲ Cells divide during the early stages of human development. Here we see four cells, soon there will be eight, and so on....

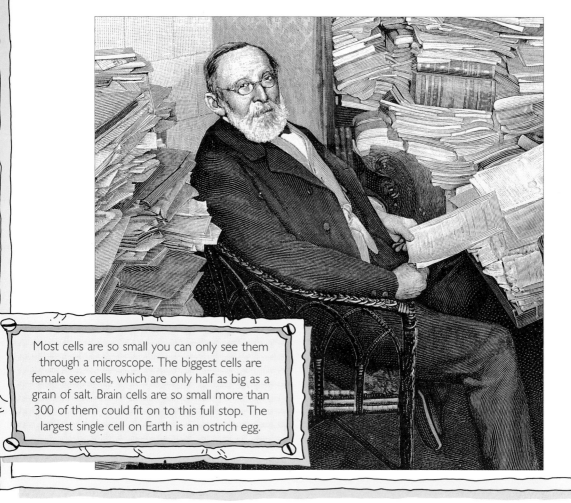

Most cells are so small you can only see them through a microscope. The biggest cells are female sex cells, which are only half as big as a grain of salt. Brain cells are so small more than 300 of them could fit on to this full stop. The largest single cell on Earth is an ostrich egg.

The sphygmomanometer

Etienne-Jules Marey FRANCE 1860

In 1628, William Harvey noticed that when an artery is cut, the blood spurts out as if under pressure. Blood pressure can be felt in the beat of your pulse (see page 24). In 1835, Julius Hérisson invented a sphygmomanometer which transferred the beat of the pulse to a narrow column of mercury. As the pulse beat, the mercury bobbed up and down. For the first time, doctors had an instrument for measuring pulse and blood pressure without opening up an artery. But it was difficult to use, clumsy and inaccurate so other scientists came up with better designs. In 1860, Etienne-Jules Marey developed the best of all. It magnified the movement of the pulse and drew a trace of it onto paper wrapped around a drum. It could also be carried from place to place. Marey used it to study irregular heartbeats.

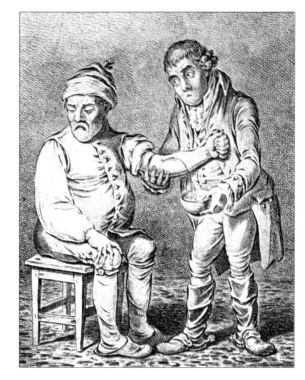

▶ A sphygmomanometer measures blood pressure using a column of mercury, in the same way that a barometer measures atmospheric pressure.

The sphygmomanometer which doctors use today was invented in 1896 by the Italian scientist Scipione Riva-Rocci. It has an armband which can be inflated with air to cut off the blood supply. The doctor listens to the pulse beat through a stethoscope and reads the pressure on a dial.

The dental drill

George Fellows Harrington

UNITED KINGDOM 1864

Filling a tooth saves it from being pulled out. The dentist drills away the rotten part of the tooth and fills it with a mixture of metals or chemicals that are hard-wearing. No filling, however, is as hard-wearing as your own healthy teeth.

John Greenwood was dentist to George Washington, the first president of the United States. He made some false teeth for Washington out of elephant's tusk and drilled his other teeth with a contraption he adapted from his mother's spinning wheel. Greenwood tapped a foot pedal to operate the drill. His invention did not catch on, however. Dentists continued to use drills that were operated by turning a handle. The fact that the first anaesthetics were used by dentists (see page 35) shows how painful early drills and tooth extractions were.

In 1858, George Harrington invented the first drill powered by a motor. The drill was attached to a clockwork device which the dentist had to hold in his hand. Other motor drills followed, some powered by electric motors, some by pneumatic. Today's drills work at high speeds with a jet of cold water to stop them getting too hot. Local anaesthetics mean that the patient feels almost no pain.

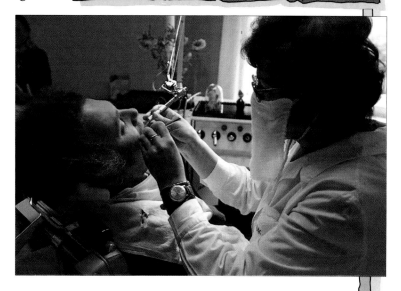

▲ Today's dental equipment uses the latest technology. Here, an ultrasound probe breaks up plaque using high frequency sound waves.

▼ The old ways of treating tooth decay were very basic and very painful!

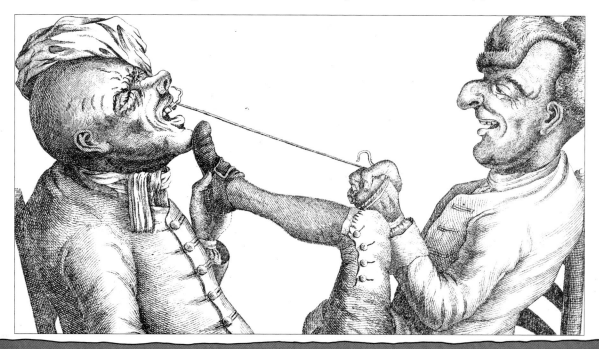

Antiseptic techniques

Joseph Lister United Kingdom 1865

In the 1860s, a famous doctor remarked that English soldiers at the battle of Waterloo had a better chance of survival than someone having an operation. Wounds became infected but most doctors still thought, as Galen had, that pus was a good thing. Joseph Lister did not agree. He had read about Pasteur's work on germs and believed that germs were responsible for turning wounds septic.

In August 1865, an 11-year-old boy was taken to Glasgow Royal Infirmary where Lister was a surgeon. Lister washed the wound with a strong disinfectant called carbolic acid before he operated. The acid burned the boy's skin, but the leg healed perfectly. Had any other surgeon been in charge, the leg would have been amputated and the boy would probably have died.

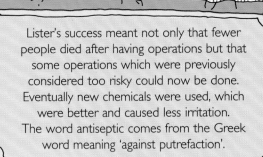

Lister's success meant not only that fewer people died after having operations but that some operations which were previously considered too risky could now be done. Eventually new chemicals were used, which were better and caused less irritation.
The word antiseptic comes from the Greek word meaning 'against putrefaction'.

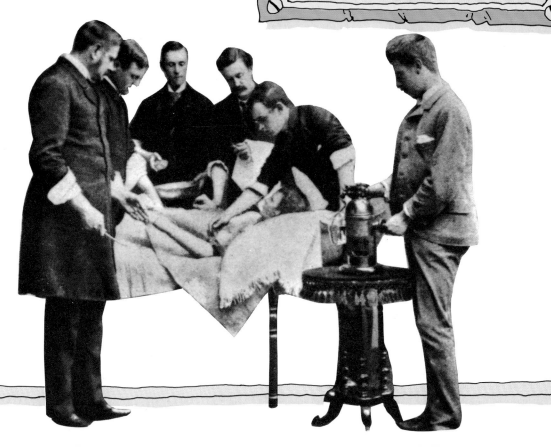

Genetics
Johann Gregor Mendel
AUSTRIA 1866

Mendel was first to study the science of 'genetics' which is the Greek word for 'give birth to' and worked out what was later known as the *Mendelian laws of inheritance*. His work helps us understand Darwin's theories of natural selection and survival of the fittest in evolution.

Mendel was living as an Augustinian monk in Brno when he became interested in Virchow's theory that certain characteristics of plants are passed on from one generation to the next. Between 1856 and 1863, Mendel planted thirty-four different kinds of pea plant and noted the differences between them, such as height, shape of seed and the colour of the flower. He made sure that no insects reached the plants so that no pollen from outside the experiment was brought in. Then he noted what sort of plants the seeds grew into. He found

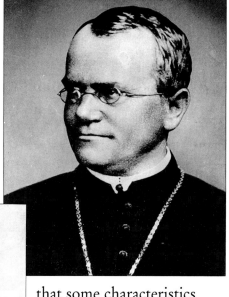

that some characteristics occur more often than others and he called these 'dominant' characteristics. Mendel believed that all characteristics were passed on from plant to plant as particles. He realized that each plant received two of each kind of particle, one from each parent. Today, we know that Mendel's particles are really genes. Mendel published his work in a botanical magazine, but it was ignored by other scientists until sixteen years after his death.

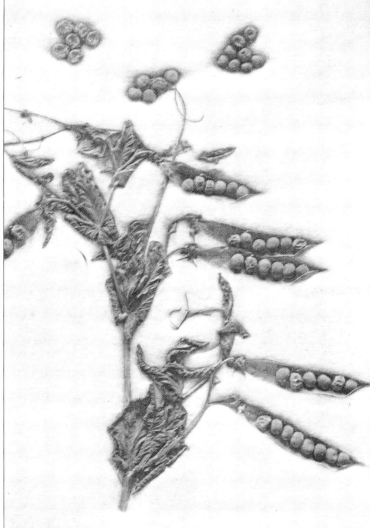

◀ This plant was produced when a yellow wrinkled pea plant was crossed, or bred, with a green round pea plant. As you can see, the peas in the pods are a mixture of round green peas and yellow wrinkled ones.

The medical thermometer

Thomas Clifford Allbutt UNITED KINGDOM 1867

If you are ill today, one of the first things a doctor does is take your temperature. The first thermometer was invented by Galileo in the sixteenth century, but it took nearly 300 hundred years for a thermometer to be designed which could easily and reliably be used by doctors. In 1714, Gabriel Fahrenheit developed a mercury thermometer with a scale fixed by the freezing point of water and the temperature of the human body. A Dutch doctor used it to investigate fever cases, but the thermometer was still too big and slow to be of use to most doctors. Then, in 1867, Allbutt devised a thermometer which registered temperature quickly and accurately and was only fifteen centimetres (six inches) long. Unfortunately, Allbutt's thermometer came too late to help Carl Wunderlich. In 1868, this German professor published *The Temperature in Diseases*. It recorded information from 25,000 patients whose temperature he had taken with a thermometer which was twice as big as Allbutt's and took twenty minutes for the temperature to register!

The mercury in medical thermometers is dangerous if the glass is broken, so a new thermometer made out of a strip of plastic can be used for babies and young children. Normal body temperature is about 37° centigrade (98.4° Fahrenheit).

▶ A nurse uses a medical thermometer take this person's temperature. Mercury is stored in the 'bulb' at the end, and when it is heated it expands up a very, very narrow glass tube, so even a small change in temperature will cause quite a large movement of mercury up the tube. The thermometer then has to be shaken to force the mercury back into the bulb.

Cancer
Wilhelm Waldeyer-Hartz
GERMANY 1867

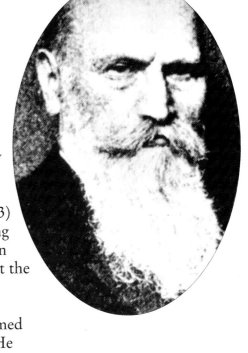

In the late eighteenth century, John Hunter put forward the idea that a substance called 'blastema' formed into tissue and was necessary for the body to repair itself. However sometimes, he said, blastema could grow when it was not needed, causing cancer. Later, Rudolf Virchow (see page 43) discovered that cells were the body's basic building blocks, not blastema, and that tumours arose when cells continued to divide when they shouldn't. But the scientist who really put the study of cancer on a modern footing was Wilhelm Waldeyer-Hartz.

In 1867, Waldeyer-Hartz wrote that cancer formed when normal cell division became uncontrolled. He also said that secondary tumours formed when a cancer cell moved in the blood and lodged in a new site. He realized therefore that the best hope of curing cancer is to detect and treat it at a very early stage. This discovery was particularly useful when treatments such as radiotherapy (see page 67) and chemotherapy (see page 72) became available.

▼ This is a sample of blood seen under a microscope. This person is suffering from cancer of the blood, which is called leukaemia.

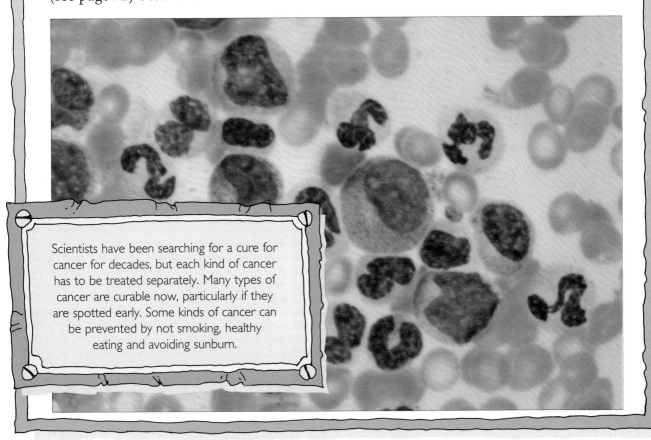

Scientists have been searching for a cure for cancer for decades, but each kind of cancer has to be treated separately. Many types of cancer are curable now, particularly if they are spotted early. Some kinds of cancer can be prevented by not smoking, healthy eating and avoiding sunburn.

OUT OF THE ASYLUM

Hypnosis
Jean Martin Charcot
FRANCE 1872

In the nineteenth century, most mentally ill people were locked away in huge asylums, where they were often neglected and ill-treated. Some doctors considered that these people were like machines that had gone wrong and tried to cure them by such methods as spinning them on a chair so fast that they fainted or pouring water over them.

Charcot, however, thought that there was a physical cause for mental disorders. He was particularly interested in hysteria, where the patient shows physical symptoms, such as paralysis, which have no physical cause. Charcot tried treating these patients with magnetism and metals but then he turned to hypnosis. He found that many hysterics could be cured by hypnotic suggestion and gave public demonstrations and lectures. He thought that only hysterics, or potential hysterics, could be hypnotized.

When a person is hypnotized he or she is totally under the control of the hypnotist. The hypnotist can then make suggestions that the patient acts on but does not remember after coming out of the hypnotic trance. Hypnotherapy can be used today to ease 'exam nerves', cure phobias (such as fear of heights or spiders) and to help people to manage pain.

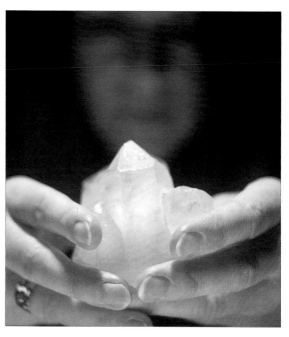

▼ Charcot demonstrates his hypnotic treatment for hysterics during one of his lectures.

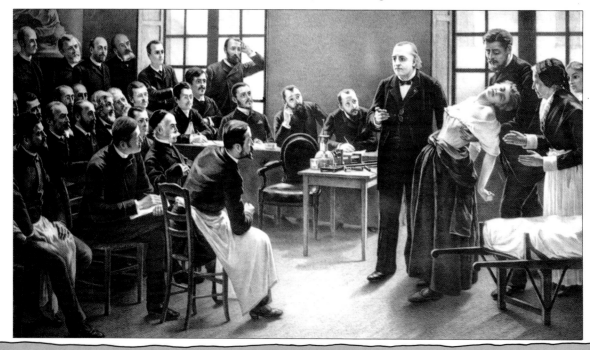

50

Leprosy

Gerhard Hansen NORWAY 1873

Leprosy is a disfiguring disease which was once common all over the world and is even mentioned in the Bible. Victims develop sores and ulcers and may become crippled. Children are most liable to catch the disease which can take two to seven years to show itself.

Hansen began studying leprosy in 1868. The disease often affected several people in a family and many doctors wondered if it was hereditary. When Hansen examined the case histories of several victims, however, he noticed that the disease died out whenever the family broke up and lived apart. Leprosy could not be inherited, so, following Pasteur's discoveries (see page 42), Hansen looked for a germ. In 1873, he spotted the bacterium *Mycobacterium leprae* which he was sure caused the illness. Although he couldn't prove the link, Hansen did persuade the government that leprosy was catching and lepers should be isolated.

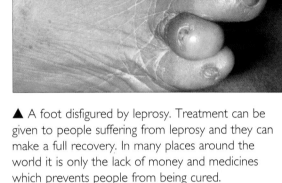

▲ A foot disfigured by leprosy. Treatment can be given to people suffering from leprosy and they can make a full recovery. In many places around the world it is only the lack of money and medicines which prevents people from being cured.

A cure for leprosy had to wait until the discovery of sulphanilamides (see page 79). The bacteria are difficult to kill and need long periods of treatment with several different drugs. There are still between ten and fifteen million lepers in the world today, mainly in tropical countries in Africa, Asia and Latin America.

◄ This man is being looked after in a leper colony in the Philippines. Colonies like this were set up because leprosy is catching. But after just a few months of treatment it should be possible for him to return to his family.

Safe vaccination

Louis Pasteur FRANCE 1881

Pasteur had proved that disease is caused by bacteria (see page 42), and Koch had identified many particular bacteria, but one question still remained: how could disease be controlled? Jenner (see page 28) developed a safe vaccine for smallpox by using a milder, similar disease, but Pasteur went on to produce safe vaccines from the disease itself.

In 1879, he had made a lucky discovery. Chickens injected with an old culture of cholera did not develop the disease. When he reinjected them with a new culture they still remained healthy. Pasteur experimented with different ways of producing a weak culture of a bacteria. Then, in 1881, he injected twenty-four sheep, one goat and six cows with a weak culture of anthrax bacteria. Two weeks later, he injected

them and an unvaccinated group with a full dose of anthrax. Only two days later, all the unvaccinated animals had died, but the vaccinated group were still healthy. Pasteur went on to develop vaccines against other animal diseases.

Pasteur's most spectacular success was in developing a cure for rabies. Anyone bitten by an infected animal had, until this time, died of the disease . He used it to treat a 9-year-old boy who had been bitten by a rabid dog. After that, people flocked to Pasteur for treatment.

▼ Vaccinations are often made from small doses of the disease itself. Today, we are all vaccinated against a variety of diseases, such as, diphtheria, tetanus, measles, mumps and polio.

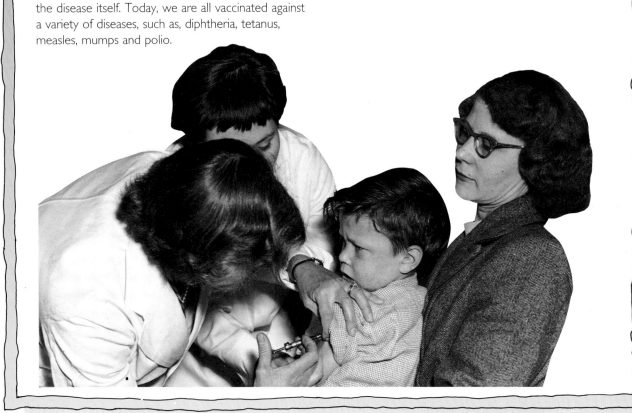

Enzymes
Wilhelm Friedrich Kuhne
GERMANY 1883

The discovery of enzymes grew out of an interest in brewing beer. In 1833, Jean-Francois Persoz discovered that it was not the malt that made the beer ferment into alcohol, but a substance secreted by the malt which was responsible for the transformation. He called the substance 'diastase'. In the next twenty years, several other similar substances were discovered.

In 1878, the German scientist Wilhelm Kuhne named these substances 'enzymes'. He worked for Claude Bernard (see page 41) and he discovered that digestion as well as brewing relies on enzymes. In 1883, Kuhne discovered that the pancreas secretes trypsin, a substance needed to break down protein.

Enzymes are themselves proteins. Each cell in the human body contains about 3,000 enzymes. They make it possible for chemical reactions to occur in the body's cells, not just for digestion but for respiration (see page 27) and other processes as well. Enzymes allow these reactions to take place at normal body temperatures. Without them, your body temperature would have to rise to 300 degrees centigrade to digest food!

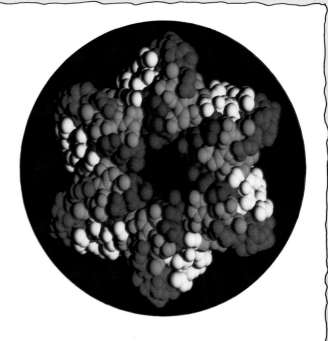

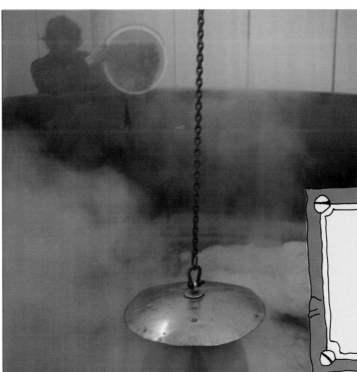

▲ A computer map of an enzyme.

◀ Adding yeast (an enzyme) is vital to the process of beer-making and distilling all kinds of alcohol. The yeast causes a chemical reaction to take place whereby most of the sugar in the mixture turns to alcohol – this process is called 'fermentation'.

Enzymes are catalysts. That means that they have to be present for a chemical reaction to take place, but they are not themselves changed in the reaction. A chemical reaction is one in which a substance changes or combines with another substance. Burning and cooking are examples of chemical reactions.

Safer surgery

William Stewart Halsted

UNITED STATES 1889

William Halsted was Surgeon-in-Chief and Professor of Surgery at Johns Hopkins Medical School for thirty-three years. He introduced many new techniques and training methods that made surgery safer for his patients. Following Lister's work with antiseptics (see page 46), Halsted made all his nurses and doctors wash their hands and arms in a sterilizing solution of mercuric chloride. In 1889, one of his nurses, Caroline Hampton, complained that the chemicals irritated her skin. Halsted asked the Goodyear Rubber Company to make her some special, thin rubber gloves. They were so successful that Halsted ordered rubber gloves for the rest of his staff and, before long, they were used in operating theatres across the world. Although Halsted was addicted to cocaine and then to morphine, he was a very careful surgeon who made sure his operations cut and injured the patients as little as possible, so that they recovered more quickly.

Today rubber gloves are used widely throughout the medical profession. Since it became known that HIV (see page 107) can be transmitted in the blood, dentists, ambulance workers, clinic nurses and many others wear rubber gloves when attending any patient.

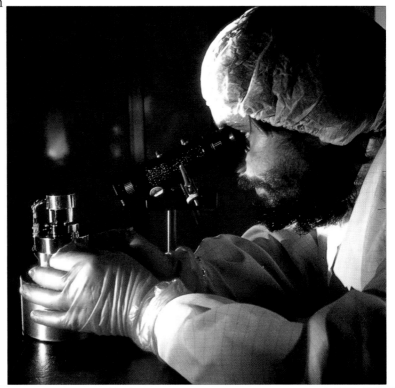

▶ Surgeons and scientists wear rubber gloves to prevent the transfer of disease. In addition to rubber gloves, doctors today wear special clothing and masks for surgery, and all the equipment used in the operating theatre is sterilized to kill any germs that could infect the patient.

BACTERIA-EATING CELLS
White blood cells
Elie Metchnikoff FRANCE 1892

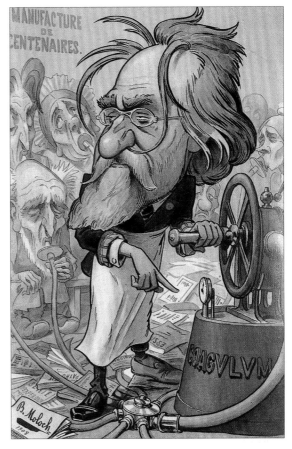

Although Pasteur (see page 52) had shown how to immunize people and animals against some diseases, the question of why immunization worked remained unanswered. Elie Metchnikoff helped to answer this question by showing how the body protects itself against disease. He put forward the idea that there are special cells in the blood which attack foreign matter which gets into the blood from outside the body. He called these cells 'phagocytes', which means 'cell-eaters' and he showed that these large white blood cells destroyed bacteria. When infection strikes the body, the number of these white cells increases.

As well as identifying many bacteria, Robert Koch identified smaller white cells called 'lymphocytes'. He also found that large white cells in vaccinated animals work better than those in unvaccinated animals. It became clear that several kinds of cells work together to form the body's immune system.

There are several kinds of white blood cell. They move along the sides of blood vessels, and when they come to a bacterium or a solid particle they flow and surround it and slowly destroy it. Sometimes the bacteria destroy the white cell, but most bacterial invasions are beaten before they cause illness.

◄ An electron microscope image showing a human white blood cell (blue) and its nucleus (orange) and the bacterium (red) that it has attacked and surrounded. When a bacteria or particle has been surrounded or 'ingested' it becomes completely harmless.

Psychoanalysis

Sigmund Freud and Josef Breuer AUSTRIA 1895

In 1881, Freud became fascinated by one of Breuer's patients, whom they later wrote about as Anna O. She suffered from several hysterical symptoms including paralysis of arms and legs, and problems with seeing, speaking and memory. Under hypnosis, Breuer asked the patient, when she first experienced each symptom. As she remembered the upsetting events connected with each, the symptoms disappeared one by one. Freud and Breuer published their findings about what Anna O called the 'talking cure' in 1895.

Freud went on to develop a better way of tracing the hidden problems that can cause emotional disturbance. By relaxing on a couch and talking about whatever they wanted to, his patients gradually came to terms with wishes and past events which they had previously found too disturbing. Freud said that it was these hidden wishes and memories, buried in the unconscious part of the mind, which made the patient ill or unhappy. Freud called his treatment 'psychoanalysis'.

▼ Freud's study in London containing the 'couch' that patients would lie on while they discussed their problems and dreams. Freud believed the purpose of psychoanalysis was to explore the 'inner self'.

Freud said that dreams can sometimes show what is hidden in the subconscious. The dream does not directly contain the event or forbidden wish, but changes it to protect you from its true meaning.

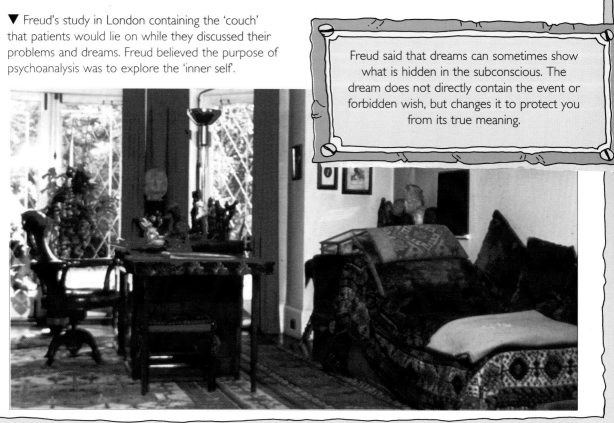

X-rays
Wilhelm Konrad Röntgen
GERMANY 1895

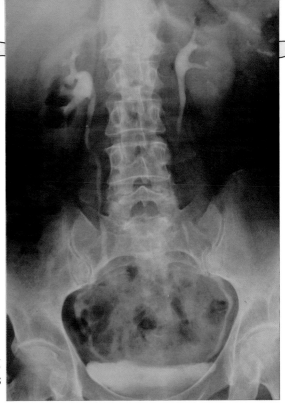

Röntgen discovered X-rays by accident when he was studying cathode rays by passing an electric current through a glass tube. Although the tube was wrapped in cardboard, a piece of photographic paper which happened to by lying nearby glowed every time the current flowed. Something, not the cathode rays, must have been passing through the cardboard and affecting the paper. Röntgen called the unknown rays 'X-rays'.

He found that they could pass through a 1,000-page book, wood and rubber, but not through lead. He held up a small piece of lead in front of the rays to make sure. The shadow of the lead appeared on the screen and so did the shadow of his hand with the outline of his bones! As soon as Röntgen published his discovery at the end of 1895, the newspapers took up the story and Röntgen became famous.

X-rays have transformed medicine. At first, they were used only to show up the bones but later, with the help of special dyes, defects in the organs were spotted too.

Some people were suspicious of X-rays at first. They were worried that 'Peeping Toms' would use them to see through their clothing. A London company put their minds at rest by advertising their new range of 'X-ray-proof' underwear.

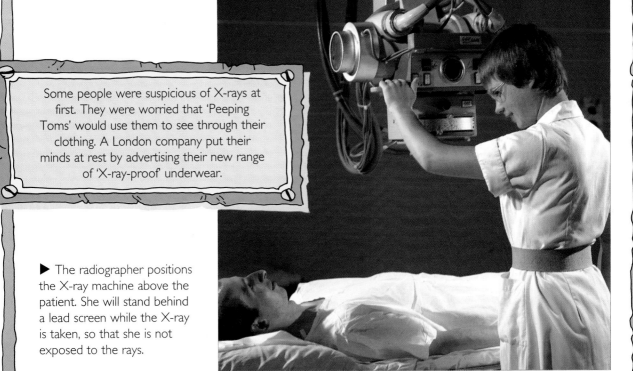

▶ The radiographer positions the X-ray machine above the patient. She will stand behind a lead screen while the X-ray is taken, so that she is not exposed to the rays.

57

A LOCK AND A KEY

Antibodies

Paul Ehrlich GERMANY 1897

Ehrlich found that when a poison, or toxin, is introduced into the body, the body makes its own antitoxin which locks onto it and destroys it.

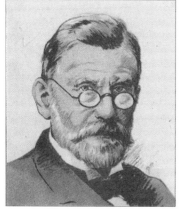

These antitoxins are called 'antibodies'.

Ehrlich was trying to solve the problem of producing a reliable vaccine for diphtheria. Diphtheria toxin can quickly lose its power, leading to very different amounts of antitoxin. Ehrlich pointed out that each molecule of toxin combines with a set amount of antitoxin, giving a standard of measurement. He said that the connection between the antitoxin and toxin was rather like a lock and a key. The antitoxin blocks the toxin. The body produces extra antitoxins, or antibodies that remain in the blood ready to fight any further invasions of that toxin, or disease. Ehrlich published his findings in a paper in 1897, laying the basis of modern immunology.

▼ Computer graphics model of an antibody (green) attacking a disease (orange). Antibodies are proteins which are carried in the blood so that they can travel to where ever they are needed in the body and fight infection.

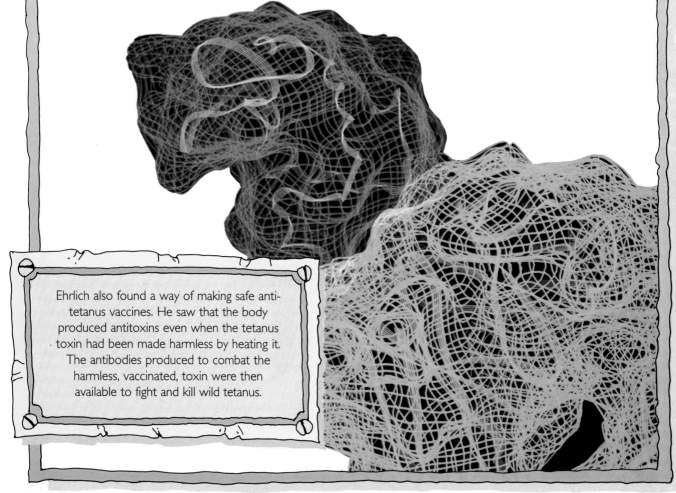

Ehrlich also found a way of making safe anti-tetanus vaccines. He saw that the body produced antitoxins even when the tetanus toxin had been made harmless by heating it. The antibodies produced to combat the harmless, vaccinated, toxin were then available to fight and kill wild tetanus.

58

Malaria

Ronald Ross UNITED KINGDOM 1897

Malaria is still one of the world's biggest killers. The word malaria means 'bad air' and even the Romans realized that certain swamps were places to avoid. But it is not the air which contains the disease, but the mosquitoes which breed in stagnant water. Ronald Ross suspected as much in 1892.

A small parasite, about the size of a red blood cell, had been discovered in malaria victims. How did it get there?

Ross managed to trace the life history of the parasite. It begins in the stomach of a mosquito and, as it breeds, its offspring invade the insect's salivary glands. Whenever the mosquito bites someone, it transfers the parasites in its saliva into the person's blood. It may be weeks later before the person is hit by the characteristic fever and shivering of malaria. The fever passes only to return again and again. Ross's work did not cure the disease, but, once the cause was understood, people could try to destroy the mosquitoes in the swamps where they breed. Malaria has mostly been wiped out from cities and towns, but still thrives in many country areas, particularly in Africa, Latin America and south-east Asia.

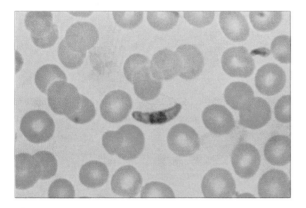

▲ The malaria parasite (purple) can be seen in the centre of this photo taken down a microscope. The disc shapes are red blood cells. 200 million people worldwide develop malaria every year.

▼ The mosquito pierces the human skin with its proboscis. It is only the female that bites to take blood, she needs it for the healthy development of her eggs, and so only the female can pass on malaria.

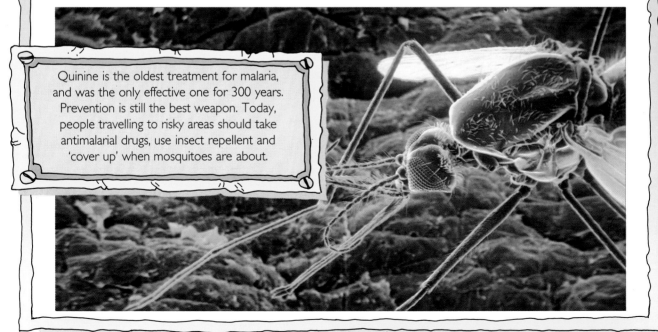

Quinine is the oldest treatment for malaria, and was the only effective one for 300 years. Prevention is still the best weapon. Today, people travelling to risky areas should take antimalarial drugs, use insect repellent and 'cover up' when mosquitoes are about.

TYPHOID MARY

Typhoid
Almroth Wright
UNITED KINGDOM 1898

The usual sources of typhoid are infected drinking water or food that have been handled by someone suffering from, or carrying, the disease. Today, typhoid can be cured by antibiotics.

When the Crimean War was fought in the 1850s, ten times as many soldiers died from typhoid as from battle wounds. Typhoid causes high fever and bleeding in the gut, and is highly infectious. By 1898, Almroth Wright had developed a vaccination against typhoid, although the disease itself was still not curable. Even in the Boer War, which started the following year, five times as many soldiers were killed by typhoid as by gunshot. By World War I, however, the vaccination was being used. Of the millions of soldiers killed in the terrible conditions of the trenches, only a hundred died of typhoid.

One problem that Wright had not foreseen was Typhoid Mary. This woman was a cook who spread epidemics of typhoid wherever she went. Although she herself did not suffer from the disease, she carried it and passed it onto others in the food she prepared. When a Dr Soper finally identified Typhoid Mary, she was arrested and put in quarantine for life.

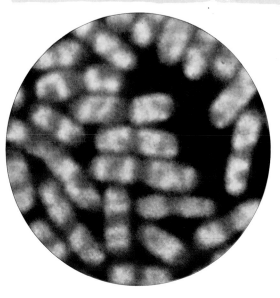

▲ A view down the microscope of typhoid bacteria enlarged about 4,000 times. The symptoms of typhoid include a high fever, a rash, chills and sweating.

▼ During the Boer War, more soldiers died from typhoid than from battle wounds.

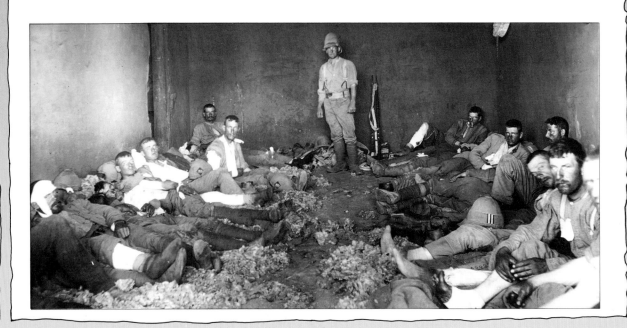

60

Aspirin

Felix Hoffman and
Heinrich Dreser GERMANY 1899

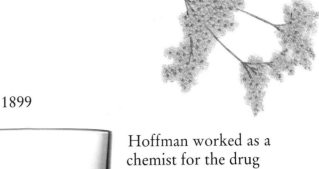

Millions of aspirins are swallowed every year to relieve headaches, toothache and other minor aches and pains. The aspirins sold today are made in the laboratory, but the first one was developed from a plant called meadowsweet which was often used in folk medicine as a painkiller.

In the 1820s, a Swiss chemist extracted salicylic acid from the meadowsweet plant. Although it was a powerful painkiller, it irritated the stomach lining, so only people who were in very great pain used it. One of these people was Felix Hoffman's father.

Hoffman worked as a chemist for the drug company Bayer. In 1895, he produced a modified version of salicylic acid and found that it not only killed the pain of his father's arthritis, but also reduced fevers and inflammation. Hoffman's colleague Heinrich Dreser experimented with Hoffman's drug which they decided to call aspirin. The next year, Bayer took out a patent on it so that no other company could manufacture it. It became the company's best-selling product.

Aspirin could have been discovered much earlier. In 1758, the Reverend Stone absentmindedly pulled off a piece of white willow bark and started to chew it. To his surprise, his rheumatic pain and fever were both relieved. Although the Reverend Stone did not know it, willow bark also contains salicin. Stone perfected his remedy and published the results, but the scientific world ignored him.

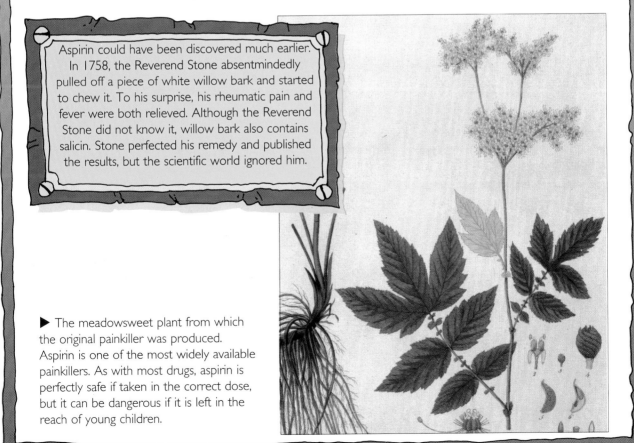

▶ The meadowsweet plant from which the original painkiller was produced. Aspirin is one of the most widely available painkillers. As with most drugs, aspirin is perfectly safe if taken in the correct dose, but it can be dangerous if it is left in the reach of young children.

Yellow fever

Walter Reed CUBA 1900

In 1900, the United States government asked Walter Reed and three other medical researchers to investigate the cause of yellow fever. In Havana, a Cuban doctor, Carlos Finlay, had been trying for nineteen years to prove that, as with malaria, mosquitoes were responsible for yellow fever, but all his experiments had failed. Walter Reed and his team agreed to test his theory.

They allowed themselves to be bitten by mosquitoes that had bitten yellow fever patients. Although they caught the disease and one of them died, it did not prove that the mosquitoes carried the disease. Only when the researchers set up experiments in isolated hospital tents were they able to prove that the mosquitoes were responsible. One group of volunteers who were isolated

Yellow fever starts with a very high temperature, followed by jaundice and, sometimes, by black vomit. Many people died from the disease, particularly in North and South America. Once Reed proved that mosquitoes carried the disease, people such as William Gorgas in Panama (see page 34) were able to prevent the illness by destroying the mosquitoes' breeding grounds.

from the mosquitoes stayed healthy, while four-fifths of a second group, who were bitten, caught yellow fever.

Today, there are still some countries where yellow fever is a problem. As a visitor to these areas you might need a certificate to prove that you have been vaccinated against the disease.

▼ In 1888 yellow fever caused widespread panic in Florida. In this picture, people are running away from a woman they suspect has the illness. It is called yellow fever, because sufferers often develop jaundice which makes the skin turn yellow.

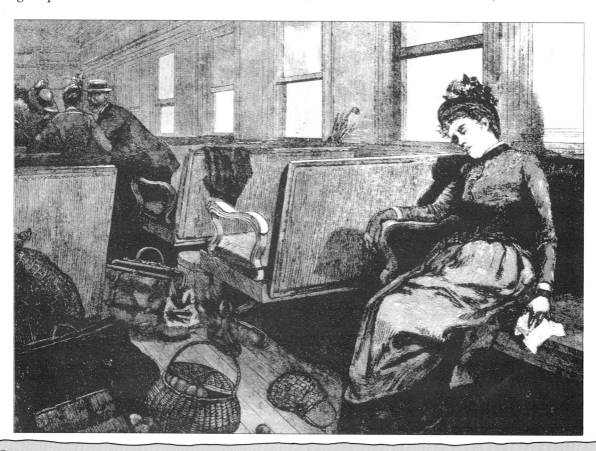

Blood groups

Karl Landsteiner AUSTRIA 1902

By the turn of the century, the prospect of having an operation was far less daunting than it had been before anaesthetics (see page 35) and antiseptics (see page 46) were invented. Yet the problems of giving blood transfusions (see page 32) were still unsolved, until Karl Landsteiner decided to investigate.

He took blood samples from himself and five of his colleagues and mixed together all of the thirty possible pairs. Some samples mixed successfully, but others produced the blood clumping that had been found with transfusions. Landsteiner then realized that the samples were not all the same. Two had a substance called an 'antigen' attached to the surface of the red blood cells, and he labelled these 'A'. Two others had a different antigen and he labelled them 'B'. Only samples with the same antigen mixed together. His own blood mixed with both A and B and Landsteiner labelled this 'O', or 'nil antigens'. He later found that another group of people have both A and B antigens, this blood is called 'AB'. At last, blood could be safely transfused.

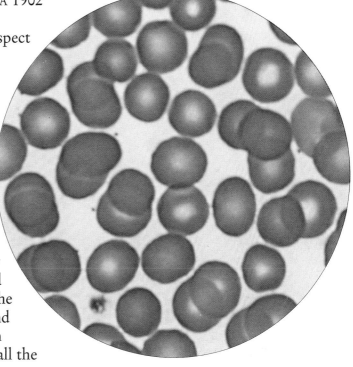

▲ Red blood cells under the microscope. All blood cells look the same, so they must be tested to see which blood group they belong to.

▼ Below, blood samples are ready to be tested.

Only compatible blood groups can be mixed together without clumping. If you have group AB blood, you can accept blood from any group. If you have group O blood, you can only receive group O blood, although you can give blood to all the other groups.

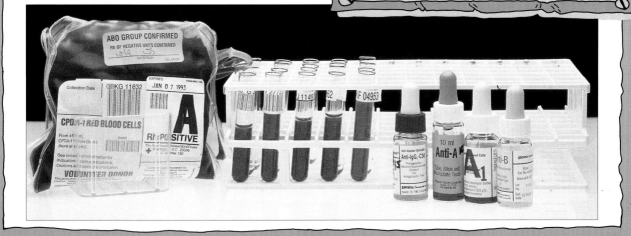

Sleeping sickness
Aldo Castellani and David Bruce UGANDA 1902

Sleeping sickness had been known in Africa since prehistoric times, but the first written account was made by an Arab traveller, Ibn Khaldun, in the fourteenth century. Victims are so lacking in energy they can easily starve to death. The chief of one tribe that Ibn Khaldun visited spent most of the time asleep and died after two years. Whole villages were killed by the disease.

In 1902, the British government sent out a commission to study sleeping sickness. Aldo Castellani was one of its members. He discovered, from doing post-mortems, that many victims had an unknown parasite in their brains.

The following year David Bruce joined the team. He had already found that a cattle disease called 'nagana' was caused by a type of parasite called a trypanosome and was spread by tsetse flies. Bruce and Castellani now found that Castellani's new parasite was trypanosome, too. Bruce mapped where the tsetse fly was found and saw that the areas coincided with sleeping sickness. People were then told to keep away from these places.

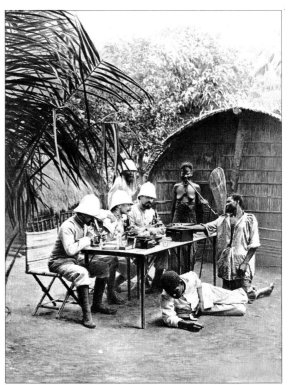

▲ French doctors at the turn of the century, studying sleeping sickness in the Congo. The tsetse fly, which passes on the disease, lives only in Africa, south of the Sahara Desert.

▶ Blood cells infected with the parasite that causes sleeping sickness.

The first drugs used to treat sleeping sickness were all compounds of arsenic, a deadly poison. Even modern drugs cannot cure severe cases. The drugs have to be taken early on in the disease for the best chance of recovery.

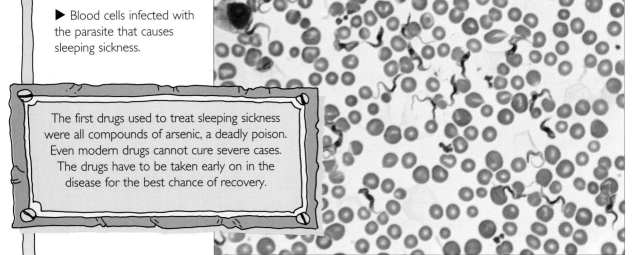

Hormones

William Maddock Bayliss and Ernest Starling UNITED KINGDOM 1902

One day in 1893, a British scientist, Edward Schafer, was measuring the blood pressure of a dog that his colleague George Oliver was walking. Oliver injected the dog with some fluid he had extracted from an adrenal gland, and asked Schafer to measure the dog's blood pressure again. It had shot up, almost to the top of the scale. Oliver and Schafer did not know it, but the extract was a hormone called 'adrenalin'.

Nine years later, Bayliss and Starling injected hydrochloric acid into another dog's duodenum. They first made sure that this part of the gut was connected to the rest of the body only by blood vessels. To their surprise, the dog's pancreas began to secrete digestive juice. Bayliss and Starling realized that the secretion in the pancreas must have been triggered by a secretion from the duodenum. Chemicals which are made in one organ and travel in the blood to stimulate another organ were later called 'hormones'. Hormones control growth and many other functions of the body.

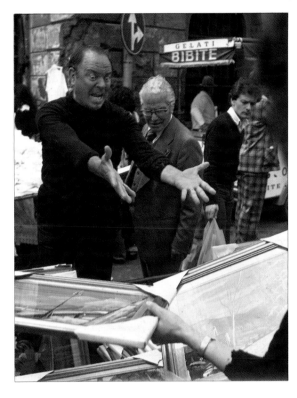

▲ When adrenalin is released in your body, it increases your heart rate and pumps more blood to your muscles, so that you are ready to stay and fight or to run away – 'fight or flight'.

▼ These vultures produce adrenalin when they are attacked by the lioness, it helps them to escape.

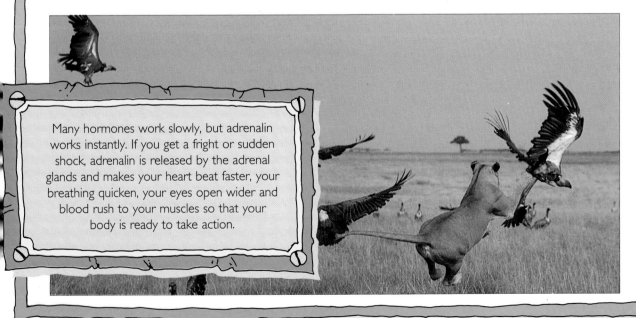

Many hormones work slowly, but adrenalin works instantly. If you get a fright or sudden shock, adrenalin is released by the adrenal glands and makes your heart beat faster, your breathing quicken, your eyes open wider and blood rush to your muscles so that your body is ready to take action.

The electrocardiograph (ECG)

Willem Einthoven NETHERLANDS 1903

In 1887, A. D. Waller showed that the working of the heart muscle generates a current of electricity, but he did not have an instrument which could record it. In 1903, Willem Einthoven made a machine which was sensitive enough to measure the electrical impulses. It was called a 'string galvanometer'. It used a fine, silver-coated quartz wire hung between the poles on an electromagnet. As electric current from the heart passed through the wire, it flickered and its shadow was recorded on a moving photographic plate. Although Einthoven realized that electrocardiographs could be used to diagnose heart disease he did not do so himself. Later scientists collected all the information needed to detect problem arteries near the heart.

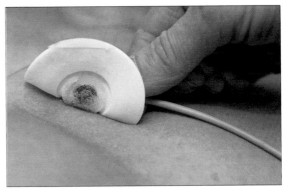

▲ A foam electrode for an ECG being attached to a patient's chest. The electrical activity of the two sides of the heart is recorded on the ECG trace.

▼ This man is being tested for cardiac fitness. To see if he has a healthy, normal heart its activity is measured during exercise, when it is working hard.

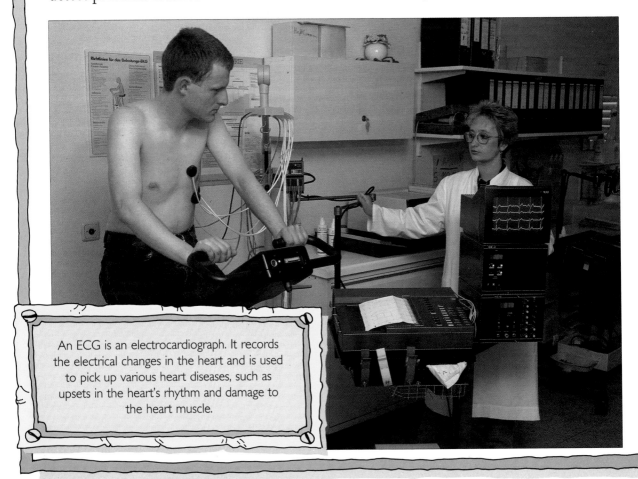

An ECG is an electrocardiograph. It records the electrical changes in the heart and is used to pick up various heart diseases, such as upsets in the heart's rhythm and damage to the heart muscle.

TREATING CANCER WITH X-RAYS

Radiotherapy

Georg Perthes GERMANY 1903

The first person to use X-rays to treat cancer was Georg Perthes. X-rays had been discovered in 1896 (see page 57), and in 1899, Pierre and Marie Curie discovered radium which is a useful source of radiation. Perthes beamed X-rays onto a malignant tumour and was delighted to find that the tumour decreased in size.

Radium, however, was a dangerous source of radiation. As well as curing cancer it could cause it, as Marie Curie herself discovered. In 1934, she died from radiation sickness as a result of her exposure to radium. Today, cobalt 60 is used as a source of radiation instead.

The first machines used for radiotherapy produced only weak beams of radiation. Most of the beams did not reach more than fifteen centimetres (six inches) inside the body, so patients whose cancers were deeper than that had to be given large doses of radiation. In the 1960s, however, better machines were developed which could direct electron beams into bones and organs without damaging the skin or surrounding tissue.

It took a long time for people to realize that X-rays had to be used sparingly. Even in the 1950s, shoe-shops used X-ray machines to check how well a shoe fitted, and doctors X-rayed pregnant women to check the development of their unborn babies. It was only in 1956 that X-rays were linked with childhood cancers.

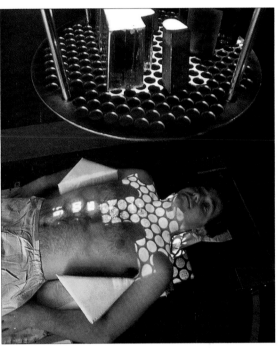

▲ A person being treated by radiotherapy. The areas that are lit will receive radiation. The radiation is targeted very accurately, so that it kills the cancerous cells, but leaves all other cells unharmed.

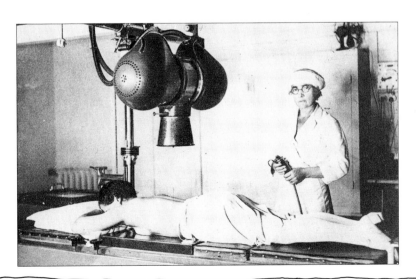

◀ An early version of the radiotherapy machine shown above. Advances in science have meant that this sort of treatment has progressed enormously over the last hundred years.

Corneal transplants

Eduard Zirm GERMANY 1906

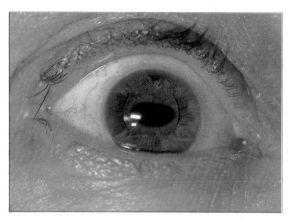

The cornea is the window between the eye and the world. If it becomes scarred, because of an accident or a disease, the person becomes blind. Today, a disease called 'trachoma' is the main cause of blindness in poor countries. The only solution is a new cornea. The first successful cornea transplant was done by Samuel Bigger just after the Napoleonic Wars. He was being held prisoner in Egypt at the time, but managed to transplant a cornea into the eye of a pet gazelle. News of Bigger's success spread and others tried to replace damaged corneas either with glass discs or with corneas taken from animals, but they were all unsuccessful.

Then, in 1906, Eduard Zirm, a German surgeon working in the

Moravian town of Olmutz, managed to attach a cornea taken from one person into another person's eye. Other surgeons tried to copy Zirm's success, but most failed. After World War II, very fine needles and even finer silk became available which allowed surgeons to stitch the corneal graft more accurately. Today, lasers (see page 97) have made the operation even easier. In fact, corneal transplants are now the most commonly performed transplant operations.

▼ Surgeons operating on the eye. A closed-circuit television shows in detail what is going on and is often used as a way of teaching students.

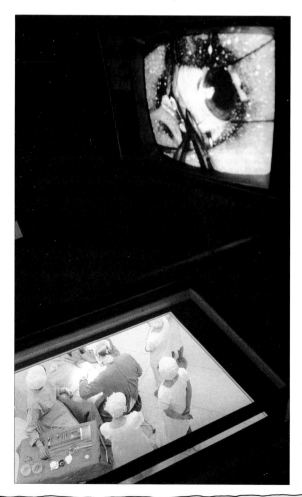

One reason why corneal transplant is so successful, is that the cornea has no blood vessels, so the transplant is less likely to be rejected by the body's immune system. The cornea does, however, have many very sensitive nerves, which protect your eye by making you blink as soon as they are triggered.

A BALANCED DIET
Vitamins
Frederick Gowland Hopkins UNITED KINGDOM 1906

In 1753, James Lind (see page 25) had shown that scurvy was caused by a lack of citrus fruit in the diet. Frederick Hopkins showed that other 'accessory food factors', as he called them, were needed too.

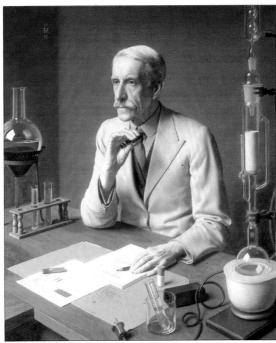

In 1906, Hopkins experimented with two groups of young rats. He fed each group on an artificial diet of casein, lard, starch, sugar and salts. This diet contained everything that was thought necessary for health and growth. One group also received a little milk and they thrived. The other group, however, did not grow. Hopkins concluded that 'astonishingly small amounts' of particular substances are needed for the body to successfully use protein and energy for growth.

Hopkins himself did not manage to isolate the particular substances and had a nervous breakdown trying. It took many years and the work of several different scientists before this was achieved. Nevertheless, in 1929, Hopkins shared the Nobel Prize for Medicine for his part in the discovery of vitamins.

▶ Fresh fruit and vegetables provide an excellent source of vitamins, and are important in a balanced diet. However, canning, pickling and over-cooking can all destroy the vitamin content of food.

The word 'vitamin' was first used by a Polish chemist, Casimir Funk, who used it as a shortening for 'vital amine'. Funk thought (wrongly) that all vitamins were compounds of ammonia (amines). But he did show how diseases such as beriberi, pellagra, rickets and scurvy were caused by a lack of particular vitamins.

The source of typhus

Charles J. H. Nicolle FRANCE 1909

Typhus is not the same as typhoid (see page 60), but the two are often confused. Patients with typhus have a high fever which can last up to two weeks and a skin rash or spots.

In 1903, Charles Nicolle was head of the Pasteur Institute in Tunis, North Africa. When he was investigating how typhus was spread from person to person, he noticed a strange thing. Before they came to hospital, typhus patients would infect other people with the disease. Once they were in a hospital ward, however, no one else caught the disease from them. So, Nicolle reasoned, the source of infection must be removed when the patient was admitted to hospital, when, like all patients, they were bathed, deloused, and their clothes disinfected. Could a body louse carry the disease?

Nicolle tested his theory. By experimenting with various animals, he managed to transmit typhus to guinea pigs, monkeys and others. He published his findings in 1909. Nicolle did much to improve the living conditions in Tunis and so reduced the disease's impact.

Typhus can now be treated with antibiotics, but epidemics of the disease still arise where people have to live together in crowded, dirty conditions in, for example, camps hastily set up for refugees fleeing from wars or famine.

▼ Charles Nicolle was able to study how typhus was passed on. He noticed that in very clean, sterile places, the disease did not occur. He worked out that the disease was carried by a body louse.

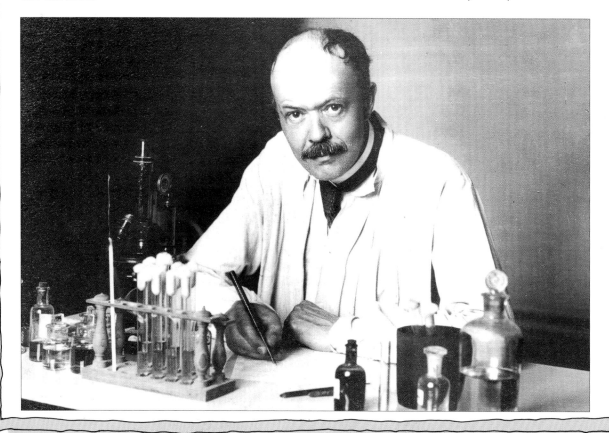

Histamine

Henry Dale UNITED KINGDOM 1910

Hay fever sufferers will know very well that pollen makes them sneeze and their eyes and nose run. One of the earliest accounts of hay fever was written by Leonardo Botallo in 1565. He called it the 'rose cold'.

In 1903, a German doctor called Wilhelm Dunbar proved that it was not the pollen itself that caused the irritation but a toxin released by the body in response to the pollen. He tried to produce an antitoxin, but it did not work. Then, in 1910, Henry Dale was studying rye poisoning when he identified a substance which he called 'histamine'. It was nearly sixteen years later before he realized that histamine produced allergic reactions. It was later found that damaged cells produced their own histamine.

It was not until the 1950s that Daniel Bovet at the Pasteur Institute in Paris developed antihistamines which work against histamine.

Asthma and eczema are also allergic conditions but, unfortunately, antihistamines do not work on them. The body always takes action against the invasion of pollen or other irritants. The problem for people with allergies is that their bodies have become very sensitive to a particular irritant.

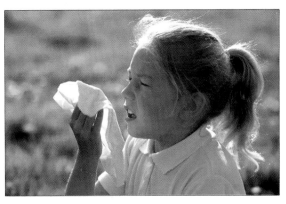

▲ Hay fever sufferers produce too much histamine, and this causes them to sneeze and their noses to run. Antihistamines are drugs which are able to control the amount of histamine produced.

▼ This bee's legs are covered in pollen after feeding from the flower. Pollen gets blown into the air and causes many people to suffer hay fever.

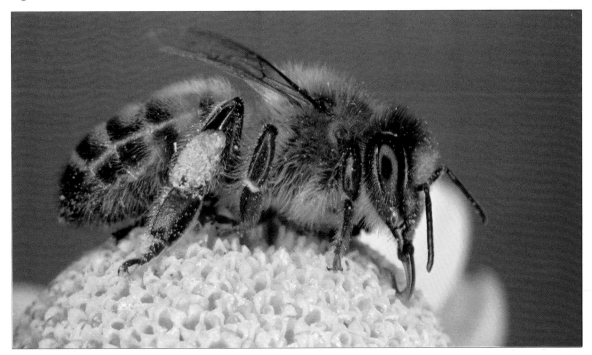

Chemotherapy

Paul Ehrlich GERMANY 1911

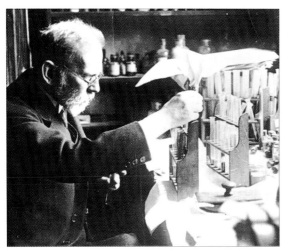

Chemotherapy is a way of treating an illness by finding a chemical which will kill the disease but not the patient. The term was first used by Paul Ehrlich, the director of an institute for researching infectious diseases and serums. In Liverpool, a synthetic (man-made) compound of arsenic had been tried against certain parasitic infections, but when Ehrlich tried to copy the results he found the disease could become resistant to the drug. He got his chemists to try making many different compounds of arsenic. Then, in 1905, another German scientist, Fritz Schaudinn, discovered the organism which caused syphilis, a disease which is transmitted by sexual intercourse. Ehrlich now tested his compounds against the new organism and was delighted to find that compound number 606 worked. He called it salvarsan and nicknamed it the 'magic bullet' as it singled out the syphilis disease. It was first used against syphilis in 1911.

Since then, scientists have been searching for a chemical which will kill cancer cells without seriously harming the patient. Thousands of compounds have to be tested before effective drugs are found.

▼ An 18-year-old patient has lost his hair after chemotherapy treatment for cancer.

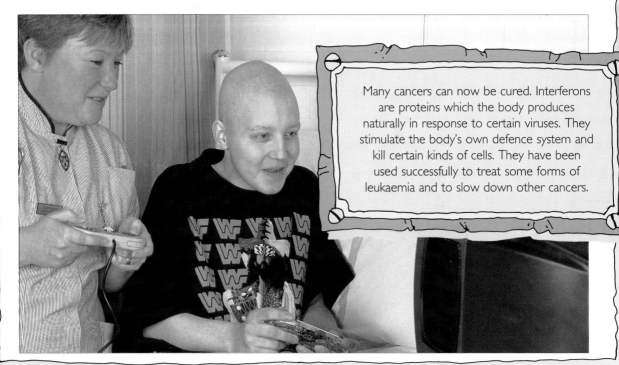

Many cancers can now be cured. Interferons are proteins which the body produces naturally in response to certain viruses. They stimulate the body's own defence system and kill certain kinds of cells. They have been used successfully to treat some forms of leukaemia and to slow down other cancers.

GIANTS AND DWARFS

The role of the pituitary gland

Harvey Cushing UNITED STATES 1912

Cushing trained as a doctor but turned to medical research almost at once. In 1908, he became interested in the functions of the pituitary gland, which is located at the base of the brain. The following year, Henry Dale extracted oxytocin from the gland. This hormone makes the uterus (womb) contract during childbirth. Cushing, however, discovered that the pituitary has a more complicated role to play.

He experimented on dogs, and then studied fifty patients whose pituitary gland either under- or over-worked. The pituitary gland controls growth and when it does not work properly it has a dramatic effect. Too much growth hormone produces very tall people and too little makes the person unusually small.

Cushing was the first person to realize that hormones are interlinked. He called the pituitary gland 'the conductor of the orchestra' because, as well as producing its own hormones, it also produces substances to control the other glands.

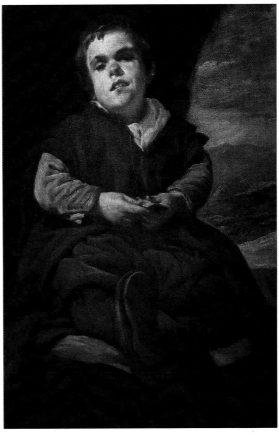

▲ A painting of Don Francisco Lezcano, who lived in the Spanish palace and was known as the Court Dwarf. Lack of growth hormone pituitary prevented him from growing to a more normal size.

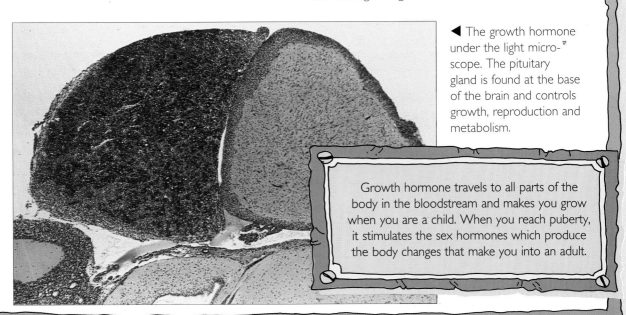

◀ The growth hormone under the light microscope. The pituitary gland is found at the base of the brain and controls growth, reproduction and metabolism.

Growth hormone travels to all parts of the body in the bloodstream and makes you grow when you are a child. When you reach puberty, it stimulates the sex hormones which produce the body changes that make you into an adult.

73

Insulin

Frederick Banting and Charles Best CANADA 1921

Diabetes is incurable, but thanks to the work of two men, Banting and Best, today's diabetics can live almost normal lives. The search to unravel the mystery of diabetes began in 1889 when two German doctors found that a dog became diabetic after they had removed its pancreas. They realized that the pancreas must secrete a hormone, but it took over thirty years before this hormone, insulin, was successfully extracted.

In 1921, Banting and Best obtained a dog's pancreas from which they managed to extract insulin uncontaminated by digestive juices. They injected it into a dying, diabetic dog. Both dog and researchers were ecstatic when, a few hours later, the dog sat up, barked and wagged its tail.

The next step was to try insulin on humans. They experimented by injecting each other, before giving the treatment to a 14-year-old boy who was dying of diabetes. Almost at once his health improved and within weeks he was completely fit and well. However, like all diabetics, he had to have regular injections of insulin for the rest of his life.

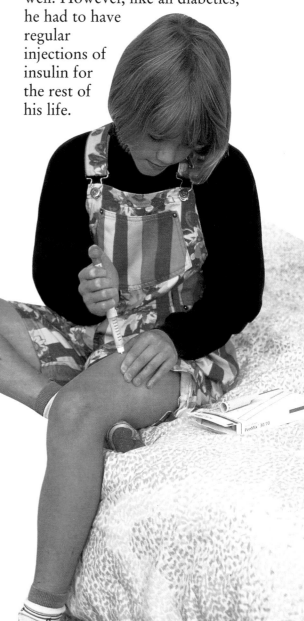

▶ A diabetic girl injects insulin into her leg. The insulin (which is normally produced in the pancreas) makes it possible for her body to break down sugar into energy.

According to a seventeenth century doctor, the quickest way to test for diabetes was to taste the patient's urine. If it was sweet like honey, the patient would surely waste away and die. Urine is still tested for excess sugars in modern-day tests for diabetes.

Electroencephalograms (EEG)

Hans Berger GERMANY 1924

The British physician Richard Caton first noticed brain waves in animals in 1875. Inspired by Wilhelm Einthoven's success with electrocardiographs of the heart (see page 66), Hans Berger decided to use a string galvanometer to measure electrical activity in the brain.

At first, he exposed the surface of a dog's brain and measured the electrical currents in the outer part of its brain. Then, he put electrodes under the scalp of humans who had had part of their skulls removed during brain operations. Finally, he was able to record brain waves through the skull and collected tracings known as 'EEGs' from his family, friends and other volunteers.

Berger first identified two different kinds of brain activity which he called alpha waves and beta waves. Later, waves were given other letters of the Greek alphabet. EEGs show different patterns of brain waves when you are thinking, resting or asleep.

EEGs are very useful in diagnosing epilepsy, a disease which involves disturbances of sensation, movement and consciousness. Anyone can have an epileptic fit, brought on by an accident, an electric shock or a high fever. People who are particularly prone to epileptic fits can now take drugs which make the fits less likely.

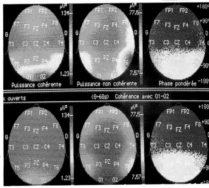

▲ Colour scans showing normal brain waves. Red and yellow indicate brain activity, blue indicates none.

▼ An EEG paper trace of an epileptic attack.

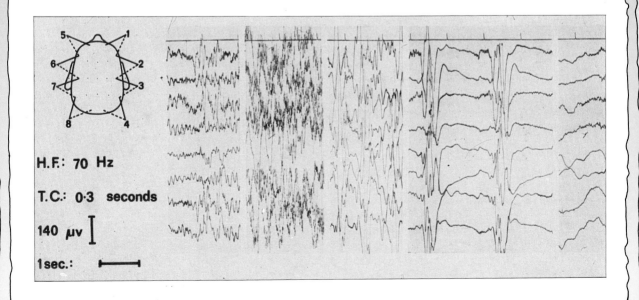

H.F.: 70 Hz

T.C.: 0·3 seconds

140 µv

1 sec.:

Penicillin

Alexander Fleming UNITED KINGDOM 1928

Howard Florey and Ernst Chain UNITED KINGDOM 1940

Alexander Fleming discovered penicillin through a lucky mistake. He left bacteria growing on culture dishes in his laboratory while he went on holiday. When he returned, three weeks later, he noticed that a mould had grown on one of the dishes and that the bacteria near the mould had all been killed. What was this powerful substance which had seeped out from the mould? Fleming called it 'penicillin' and found that it could kill many serious infections. However, because penicillin lost its power when mixed with blood in a test-tube, Fleming concluded that it wouldn't work on animals and people.

Over ten years later, in 1940, Florey and Chain tried again. They injected eight mice with a fatal dose of streptococci then gave four of them penicillin. Within a few hours, only the four mice who had been treated with penicillin were still alive and well. 'It looks like a miracle!' said Florey.

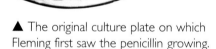

▲ The original culture plate on which Fleming first saw the penicillin growing.

▼ Fleming discovered penicillin, but it was Florey and Chain who realized its true importance.

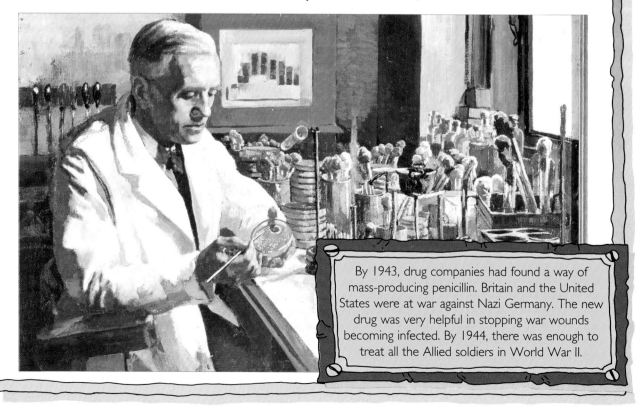

By 1943, drug companies had found a way of mass-producing penicillin. Britain and the United States were at war against Nazi Germany. The new drug was very helpful in stopping war wounds becoming infected. By 1944, there was enough to treat all the Allied soldiers in World War II.

The electron microscope

Ernst Ruska GERMANY 1928

The invention of microscopes allowed scientists like Leeuwenhoek (page 21), Bonomo (page 22) and Pasteur (page 42) to study cells, bacteria and other aspects of the way the body works. But by the late 1920s, little more could be discovered with an optical microscope.

In 1928, Ernst Ruska built a microscope which used electrons instead of light and could magnify to seventeen times life size. By 1933, he had increased the magnification to 1,200 times. Ruska found that if he passed a beam of electrons through a magnetic field they behaved as light does passing through a glass lens – they magnify the image of an object. Electrons have a shorter wavelength than light and give much greater magnification. By 1939, scientists could see not just cells, but inside the cells themselves. By 1965, the University of California was using a three-dimensional electron microscope to magnify nerves 20,000 times.

Today's electron microscopes can magnify a million times. In the 1970s, Heinrich Rohrer and Gerd Binnig developed a scanning tunnelling electron microscope which can show the structure of atoms. In 1986, when Ruska was nearly 80 years old, he shared a Nobel Prize with Rohrer and Binnig.

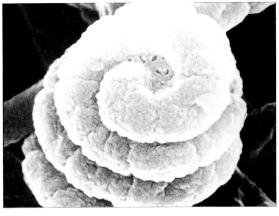

▲ A soil bacteria viewed down an electron microscope, it has been magnified 30,000 times.
▼ Using an electron microscope in the laboratory.

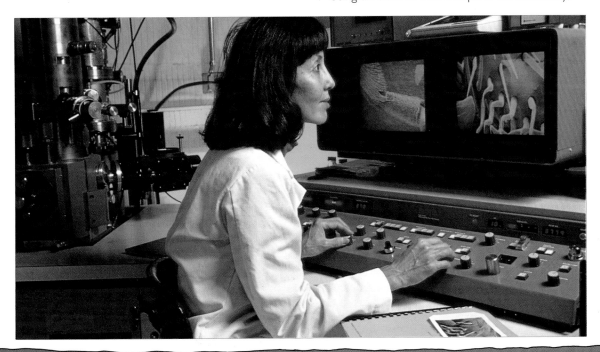

A MACHINE FOR BREATHING

The iron lung

Philip Drinker UNITED STATES 1929

Polio is a disease that can attack the nerves in the spinal cord and cause paralysis. The part of the body that is paralysed depends on which nerves are attacked. Polio can even affect a patient's ability to breathe. Lungs do not have their own muscles. They are controlled by the movement of the diaphragm, a sheet of muscle between the stomach and the lungs. As the diaphragm moves up, it pushes air out. As it moves down, air is sucked in. The nerve which controls breathing is at the very top of the neck. If this nerve was attacked by the polio virus, a patient would die. But when Philip Drinker invented the iron lung, he invented a machine that breathed for the patient. Only the patient's head stuck out of the airtight

The iron lung had a short career. Polio was brought under control in the 1950s when Salk developed a successful vaccination (see page 89). Today, there are several less cumbersome forms of respirator available to patients who need help with breathing.

iron box which was attached to a pump. As air was sucked out of the box, fresh air was drawn into the patient's lungs. When the air pressure in the box rose again, air was pushed out of the lungs. The iron lung kept many people alive. It was the first machine to take over one of the vital functions of the body.

▼ A premature baby is kept alive in a miniature iron lung. The temperature and humidity around the baby are carefully monitored and controlled.

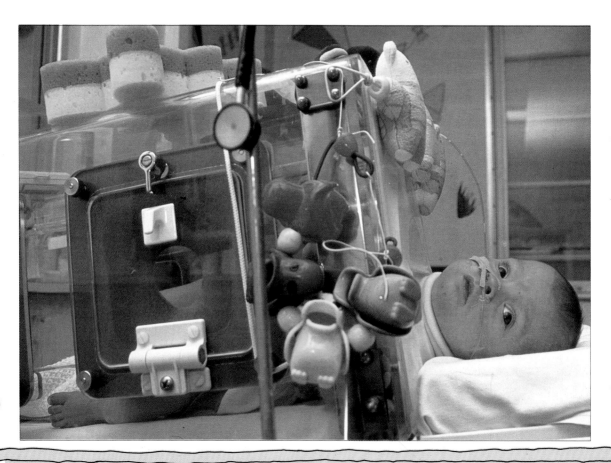

Prontosil

Gerhard Domagk GERMANY 1935

Streptococci are bacteria that can infect your throat, mouth and gut. Many people used to die from infections caused by these bacteria until Gerhard Domagk developed the drug prontosil which could kill streptococci and was the first of a family of drugs called 'sulphanilamides'.

In 1932, Domagk had discovered that a red dye killed streptococci when he injected it into infected mice. Although Domagk did not publish his findings until 1935, scientists at the Pasteur Institute in Paris heard about his discovery. They tried the same experiment and found that the drug worked on people as well as mice, although the dye turned their skin bright red. The scientists then discovered that the drug split into two parts and, luckily, the active part, sulphanilamide, was colourless. No one knows why it took Domagk so long to publish his findings, but it is likely that he knew that prontosil had already been patented as a dye. He delayed publication and thousands suffered while he tried to find a similar chemical that he could patent.

> Sulphanilamides were the best drugs for fighting bacteria until penicillin was discovered (see page 76). Sulphanilamides act not by killing the streptococci bacteria but by stopping them from multiplying. For the first time they provided a cure for diseases such as pneumonia and childbed fever.

▶ There is now a wide range of drugs available to help fight disease, but prontosil was an amazing breakthough when it was discovered – in a time when you could die from a sore throat.

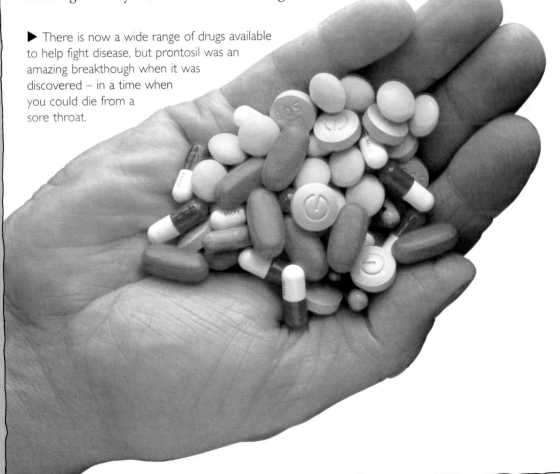

NEW HIPS FOR OLD

Hip replacement

John Wiles UNITED KINGDOM 1938

Arthritis is a painful, incurable disease which affects the joints, particularly of old people. If the hip joint is affected, the patient cannot walk, and the only treatment is to replace it with artificial materials. Today, total hip replacement is one of the most common operations.

The first hip replacement was done in 1891 by a German surgeon, Theodore Gluck. He is said to have cemented an ivory ball and socket on to the hip joint. When John Wiles performed a similar operation in 1938, he used stainless steel for the head of the joint.

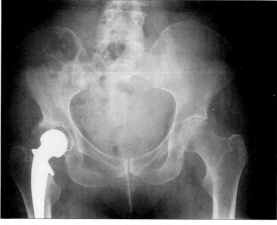

▲ An X-ray of an artificial hip joint in place. Computers are now used to design the hip joints so they exactly match the old socket. A hip joint is now expected to last for about twenty years.

Today's total hip replacements use materials developed by the British surgeon, John Charnley. He was trained both as an engineer and as a surgeon. He used a stainless steel ball and spike which fitted into an polythene cup. Both the spike and the cup were cemented in with an acrylic cement.

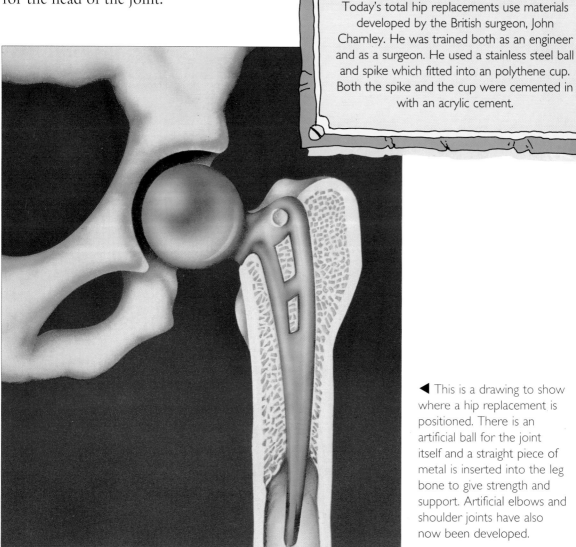

◀ This is a drawing to show where a hip replacement is positioned. There is an artificial ball for the joint itself and a straight piece of metal is inserted into the leg bone to give strength and support. Artificial elbows and shoulder joints have also now been developed.

Plastic surgery
Archibald Hector McIndoe UNITED KINGDOM 1940s

War not only kills people, it also leaves them injured and disfigured. After World War I, Harold Gillies set up a plastic surgery unit in England to treat the horrendous facial injuries that many soldiers had received. He was the first plastic surgeon to try to make his patients look as acceptable as possible. In 1932, he hired a New Zealand surgeon, Archibald McIndoe, as his assistant.

World War II brought in a new type of casualty, men who had been shot down from aeroplanes with burnt hands and faces. McIndoe transplanted skin from other parts of their bodies to cover the burnt areas. He tried to reconstruct their faces, and the men often had to undergo years of operations. One patient grumbled, 'We're not fliers any more. We're nothing but a plastic surgeon's guinea pigs!' McIndoe's patients formed a club they called the 'Guinea Pig Club'. It soon had more than 600 members from sixteen different countries. The techniques pioneered by McIndoe have since been used to help other badly burned patients.

The severity of burns depends on how deeply the skin is affected. First degree burns affect only the surface of the skin. Second degree burns affect the new, living skin underneath. Third degree burns affect the whole thickness of skin. New skin can only grow from the edges of the wound, and so with a large wound another piece of skin is 'grafted' on.

▼ Today, many people have cosmetic plastic surgery; this kind of treatment is expensive and often very painful.

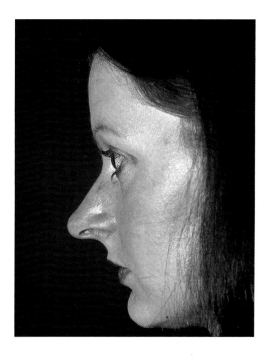

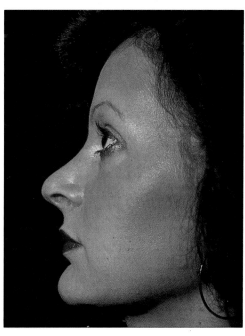

▲ This woman has had an operation on her nose to make it smaller. The top picture is 'before', the bottom one is 'after'.

Open-heart surgery

Alfred Blalock UNITED STATES 1943

In 1866, Armand Trousseau had suggested that the heart could be reached by cutting between the ribs, and this was later tried out successfully in England. Various operations were tried during the next seventy years and the success rate gradually improved. But it was not until 1944 that 'open-heart' surgery hit the headlines for the first time.

Some babies are born with only a narrow artery connecting the heart and lungs. This means that their blood does not get enough oxygen and they turn a bluish colour. There used to be no way of curing this defect, so blue babies did not live long. But Helen Taussig noticed that some babies survived longer. These babies had retained a duct between the heart and the lungs which normally closes after birth. One defect cancelled out the other. She asked Alfred Blalock if he could provide an artificial duct to do the same job in other babies. To do this, he would have to perform open heart surgery. In 1944, he successfully inserted an artificial duct into the heart of a 15-month-old blue baby.

Many 'blue babies' often have an additional heart defect. There is a communication between the left and right sides of the heart so that blood which should be sent to the lungs for oxygen is pumped back around the body. They are sometimes known as 'hole-in-the-heart' babies.

▼ To perform open-heart surgery, doctors have to make a large cut in the chest and clamps are used to hold the wound apart during the operation.

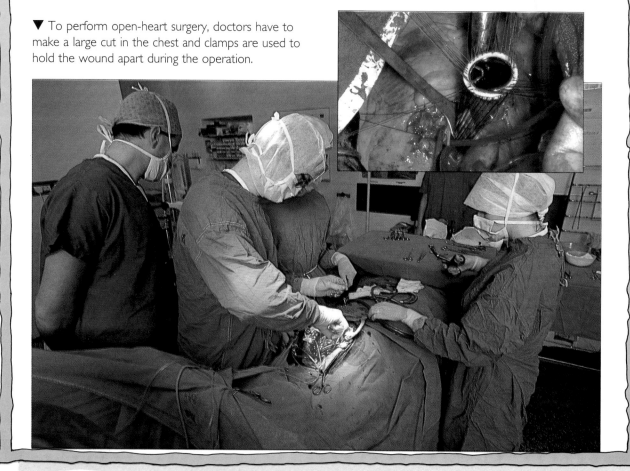

A CURE FOR TB

Streptomycin

Selman A. Waksman UNITED STATES 1943

The discovery of penicillin (see page 76) encouraged researchers to look for other wonder drugs. Could one be found to combat tuberculosis (TB), meningitis or typhoid, against which penicillin did not work? Selman Waksman decided to concentrate on a mould which produced a substance called 'streptomyces griseus'. The problem was that no two cultures of the substance were the same. Then he had some luck.

A farmer took one of his hens which was suffering from a mysterious illness to the research station at Rutgers University where Waksman worked. There, a vet took a sample from a white spot in the hen's throat. He analysed it and found it was streptomyces griseus, so sent it to Waksman for testing. To Waksman's delight, and unlike previous cultures, it killed many bacteria, including that of TB. Waksman's team turned the chicken farm upside down, before they found the soil from which the successful culture had come. When they tried the new drug on people, they found it not only cured TB, but also meningitis and even the plague.

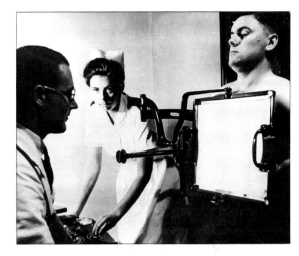

▲ Tuberculosis also used to be called consumption. It usually affects the lungs, so patients thought to have the disease have a chest X-ray, which is used to show up any infection of the lungs.

▼ A petri dish containing growths of the natural antibiotic, streptomycin, which is found in soil.

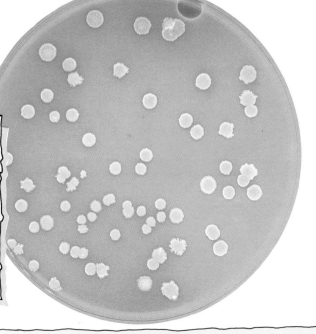

TB used to be called the 'wasting disease' because patients became very thin and weak before they died. Streptomycin alone did not win the war against TB. Millions of people still catch it every year, but vaccinations and a combination of streptomycin with other drugs has greatly reduced the number of deaths.

Kidney dialysis

Willem Kolff HOLLAND 1943

The first artificial kidney machines were only used for emergencies to keep a kidney going until it could recover itself, but, in the early 1960s, smaller machines made it possible to give a patient repeated dialysis in their own homes.

Kidneys filter the blood to remove impurities. If they fail, the impurities build up and eventually poison the body. In 1914, John Jacob Abel and a team of American scientists managed to make an artificial kidney for a dog. It was not until 1943, when Holland was occupied by the Nazis, and Europe was shattered by World War II that Willem Kolff managed to make the first kidney dialysis machine which could be used on humans. He followed the methods of John Abel, but for the tubes he used sausage casings. These were placed in a bath of sterile water. The impurities leaked from the blood into the water, through tiny holes in the sausage casing until finally the water and blood contained equal amounts of impurities, and the partly cleaned blood was returned to the body.

Kolff's machine was later improved so that the blood passed through large flat plates of cellophane. The plates were very clumsy and were later replaced by coils of cellophane tube.

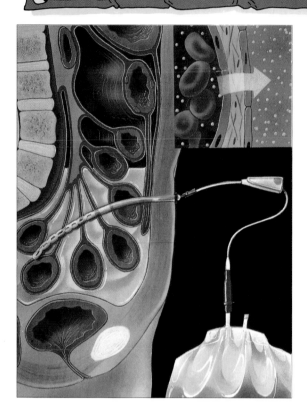

▲ This diagram illustrates peritoneal dialysis which works in the same way as kidney dialysis; fluid is introduced into the peritoneal cavity and drained out again once equilibrium has been reached.

▼ A patient receiving dialysis treatment in hospital.

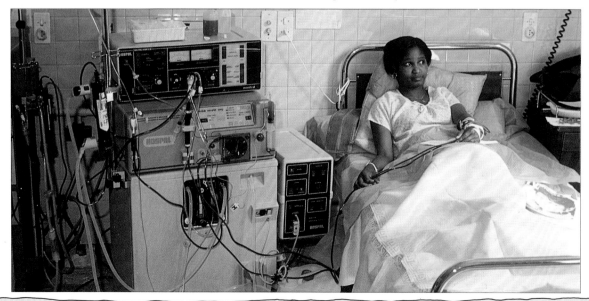

Cortisone

Philip Hench and Edward Kendall UNITED STATES 1948

Scientists were very interested in cortisone during World War II. On both sides it was thought that it helped to relieve the emotional stress known as 'battle fatigue', but no one could produce it in large enough quantities. Then, in 1944, Lewis Sarrett, an American chemist, managed to process it from the bile of cattle.

Cortisone came too late to help in the war, but Hench and Kendall decided to try it on rheumatoid arthritis sufferers. The result seemed to be miraculous and they received a Nobel Prize for their work. Cortisone reduced inflammation and allergies and was immediately prescribed for a wide range of diseases.

It was soon discovered, however, that while cortisone relieved the pain of rheumatoid arthritis, it did not stop its progress. In addition, if patients took cortisone for a long time they developed diabetes or high blood pressure, so the doses had to be carefully controlled.

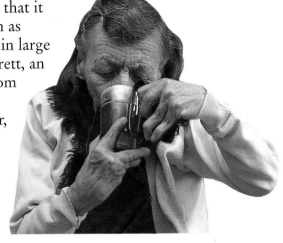

▲ Very bad arthritis can make even simple, everyday actions difficult; it most commonly affects the elderly.

A new use for cortisone was found in the 1950s, when surgeons began to carry out transplants of kidneys, hearts or skin from one person to another. Normally the body's immune system fights against anything it thinks is foreign to it, which can lead to it rejecting a transplanted organ. Cortisone helps to reduce this reaction.

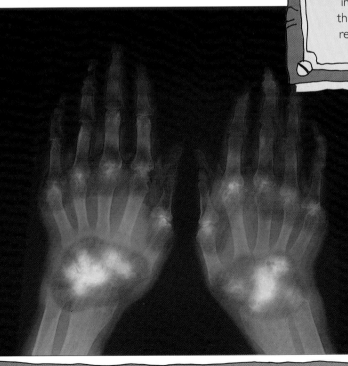

◄ This false-colour X-ray shows how the joints of an arthritis sufferer become swollen and deformed. Cortisone is used to reduce the swelling and relieve the pain.

Tranquillizers
John Cade AUSTRALIA 1949

Psychoanalysis (see page 56) works well with people who are upset and unhappy, but is much less successful in helping people with severe mental illness. John Cade wondered whether psychosis was caused by a chemical imbalance. By testing the urine of psychotic patients on guinea pigs, he stumbled on the fact that lithium, obtained from a dilute solution of uric acid, made excitable animals calm again. Cade tested it on himself and then on patients suffering from an illness called 'manic depression'. Lithium helped to make them less overexcited or 'manic', and less depressed. Cade published his results in 1949.

While Cade was working in Australia, researchers in France were looking for a drug to slow the body down. Surgeons thought that such a drug could protect their patients from shock following an operation. In 1950, Delay and Deniker produced chlorpromazine. It not only helped after surgery but also succeeded in calming mental patients. It is used today to treat schizophrenics and manic depressives.

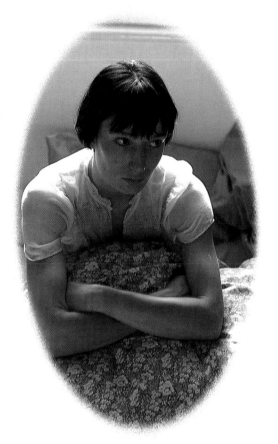

▲ Tranquillizers can help people who feel very depressed or worried, they can be used to treat mental tension without interfering with normal brain activity.

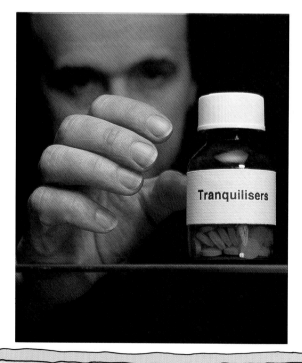

Chlorpromazine was the first drug to work directly on nerve cells and was the first true tranquilliser. It was so successful that drug companies around the world quickly developed tranquillizers not only to suit all kinds of mental disturbance but also to reduce many different types of anxiety.

◀ It is important that people only take tranquillizers when they have been prescribed by a doctor – they can become addictive if taken for long periods.

The structure of DNA

Francis Crick, James Watson and Rosalind Franklin

UNITED KINGDOM 1953

Gregor Mendel had shown that physical characteristics are passed from parents to offspring (see page 47), but no one knew exactly how. In 1944, an American scientist, Oswald Theodore Avery, suggested that DNA, which is found in the nucleus of cells, might carry genetic information. Before the theory could be proved, it was essential to discover the structure of DNA. How could one molecule carry so much information?

Many scientists took up the problem. In London, Rosalind Franklin took clear X-ray pictures of pure DNA. In Cambridge, physicists Crick and Watson formed a team. They knew that DNA contained four bases but not how they fitted together. By using just two bases, the Morse code can make all the words in the dictionary, so four bases could produce a very complicated code. Using one of Franklin's X-ray pictures, Crick and Watson built a double spiral model of a molecule which fitted all the known facts. It looked like a twisted ladder. In 1962, they and Franklin's boss (but not Franklin herself), Maurice Wilkins, received a Nobel Prize.

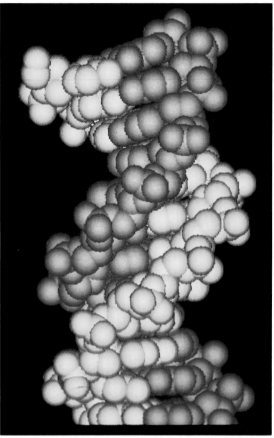

▲ The double helix shape of the DNA molecule. In cell division the DNA strand splits in two, and each half copies itself, forming two DNA molecules from one. This is how living things grow. Sometimes the DNA strands do not copy themselves exactly, and a mutation (something abnormal) is created.

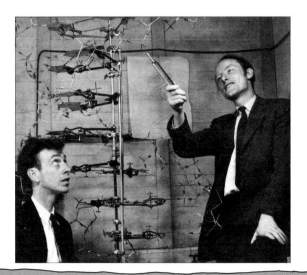

After Crick and Watson had constructed a model for DNA, biologists then tried to find out how the code it contained could produce a new, unique life. They discovered that genes are lengths of DNA which contain about 2,000 bases. The order of the bases gives the genetic code. The DNA for each human cell contains about 10,000 million pairs of bases.

The heart-lung machine

John H. Gibbon UNITED STATES 1953

In 1930, John Gibbon helped to operate on a woman who had a clot of blood blocking the artery between her heart and lungs. The woman died but her death made Gibbon determined to invent a machine that could take over the work of the heart and lungs. It took him twenty-three years.

His first machine used a hollow metal cylinder. As the cylinder spun, blood was forced onto its inner surface and oxygen was blown onto it. Unfortunately the machine could not process the blood quickly enough. Gibbon was in despair. Then his colleagues improved the design by covering the inside of the cylinder with a wire mesh that agitated the blood so that it absorbed oxygen quicker. With this improved machine, Gibbon found he could oxygenate enough blood to keep a person alive. In 1953, he used it to operate on an 18-year-old girl. The girl was on the machine for forty-five minutes and for twenty-nine minutes it took over completely the work of both her heart and lungs.

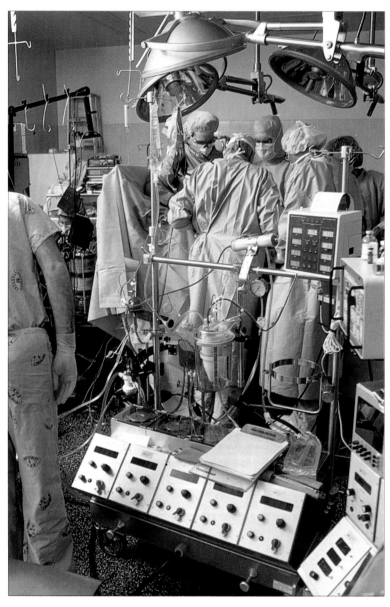

▲ During a heart transplant operation a heart-lung machine is used to keep the patient's vital body functions going. The machine pumps blood, adds oxygen to it and removes unwanted carbon dioxide.

It is very difficult to operate on a heart that is still working, but until 1953 it was impossible to stop it for more than a minute or two. The brain, or any part of the body, begins to die if it is deprived of oxygen in the blood for more than four minutes.

Polio vaccine

Jonas Salk UNITED STATES 1954

In the 1940s and 50s, parents in richer countries were very concerned by epidemics of polio which attacked school-age children. If the disease affected the spinal cord, the child could become permanently paralysed. By 1951, three different strains of polio had been identified.

Jonas Salk started work on producing a vaccine against all three strains. His first trial included his own three children. The vaccine worked, but Salk did not feel confident that it was completely safe. In 1954, a large trial went ahead, however, and the results were very successful. The children all developed antibodies to the three polio strains, and not one of those vaccinated caught the disease. When people heard the news, they sounded factory sirens and rang the church bells. By May 1955, four million American children had been vaccinated.

Salk was more cautious about his vaccine than the American people. He knew that it was not totally effective against one of the strains of polio and that children had to receive regular vaccinations to keep up their immunity.

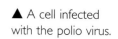

▲ A cell infected with the polio virus.

Polio was a disease that particularly affected richer countries. In poorer countries most children catch the disease from sewage when they are very young. The disease is then very mild and it gives them immunity. In places where clean water was available, older children who had no immunity caught the disease and suffered much more badly.

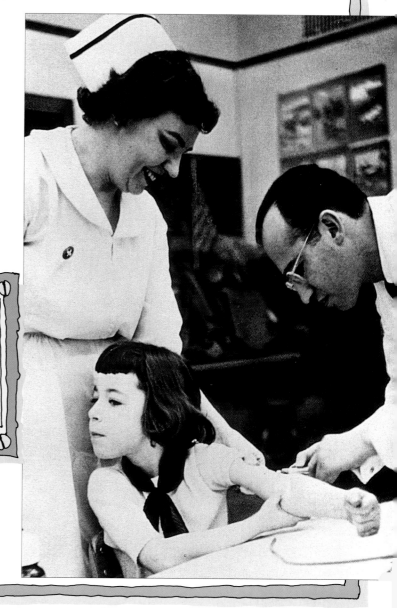

▶ Salk giving his polio vaccine to children in America. Polio used to be known as 'infantile paralysis', because of its devastating effects.

Oral contraceptives

Russell Marker MEXICO
Gregory Pincus UNITED STATES 1955

In the early 1940s, Russell Marker made a lucky discovery. He found that an extract from yams could easily be changed into progesterone, a female sex hormone. It is this hormone which controls the release of egg cells, or 'ovulation', in women. Marker set up a company to market his discovery. A sample of the company's compound was sent to Gregory Pincus, a research biologist in Massachusetts, who discovered that, when swallowed as a pill, it could prevent ovulation.

Pincus was not interested in developing birth control but Margaret Sanger (see page 33) was. She saw contraception as a way of reducing the numbers of poor people. She got money for Pincus to research 'hormonal birth control' and trials were begun first in Boston and then, in 1955, among poor women in Puerto Rico. By 1957, 'the pill' was approved in the United States as an oral contraceptive.

◀ There is a wide variety of oral contraceptives available today. The contraceptive pill contains chemicals similar to natural female hormones and, if used properly, can be about 100 per cent effective.

Oral contraceptives have provided women with a way of controlling their lives and the size of their families. However, in some cases there may be side effects. Women taking the pill are strongly encouraged not to smoke.

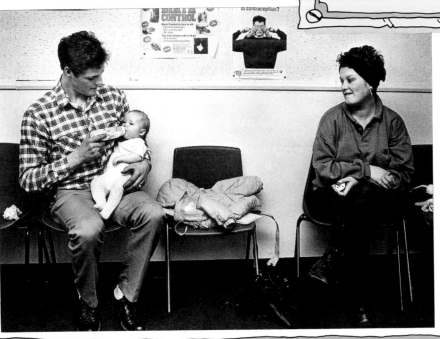

◀ There are familly planning clinics now, which give help and advice to people planning when to have their families, and help couples decide which is the best form of contraception for them.

A LENS TO COVER THE EYE

Contact lenses

Norman Bier UNITED KINGDOM 1956

The first contact lens was developed in the United States in 1887 by Louis J. Girard, but his glass lens covered the white of the eye as well as the cornea. Corneal lenses were developed by accident by an American optician. As he was making the large lens, the corneal part broke off. The lenses were still very difficult to use, even after 1936 when they were made of a lighter material called 'plexiglass'. It was not until 1956 that Norman Bier made his much smaller lenses out of a substance called 'methacrylate'. Bier's lenses were easy to put in and take out, and many people eagerly switched to using them. Nine years later, in 1965, an American company started manufacturing soft lenses, which are better for the eyes.

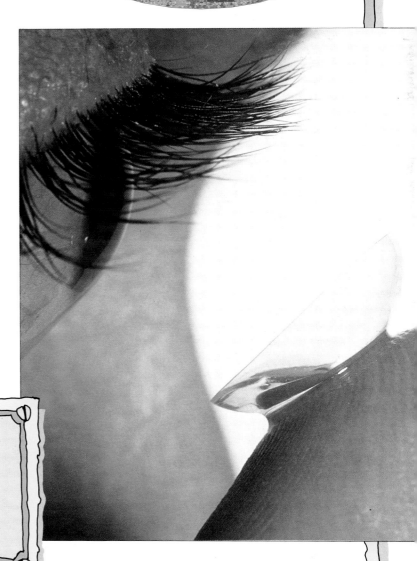

▶ A girl inserts her contact lens. An optician should be able to select a contact lens so that it fits the eye perfectly. You should not be able to feel any discomfort.

If contact lenses are not kept clean and moist they cause sore eyes and eye infections. Most lenses have to be taken out every night and soaked in cleansing solution. A new kind of permeable lens can be left in the eye for longer, but still has to be cleaned regularly and always kept moist.

Ultrasound scanning

Ian Donald UNITED KINGDOM 1957

Ultrasound is a technique used by ships to detect submarines and other underwater objects. Sonar, as it is known, uses sound waves which are so high-pitched they cannot be heard but which travel well through watery liquids. When the sounds hit an object, they send back echoes which can be converted into electrical signals and used to make a picture of the object.

Thirteen weeks after conception, a baby is properly formed but is only about six centimetres (three inches) long. Ten weeks later, the baby might survive if born, but only in an incubator. For the next fifteen weeks it grows bigger and stronger until, at about thirty-eight weeks, it is ready to be born.

To begin with, Ian Donald used ultrasound to detect stomach tumours, but by 1957 he was using it to detect problems in unborn babies. By sliding the scanner over the mother's abdomen, he could pick up a picture of the baby itself. X-rays had already done this, but doctors had come to realize that X-rays could cause childhood cancers. Donald was worried that ultrasound might have similar effects, but his fears have not been justified.

Today, ultrasound scans are used routinely to check that the foetus is growing normally. Computers are used to change the sound signals into a visual picture and the quality of the image is so good, even small abnormalities can be detected.

▼ This woman is able to see pictures of her unborn baby. The nurse may be able to tell the sex of the baby; some parents like to be told what to expect, others prefer to wait until the actual birth.

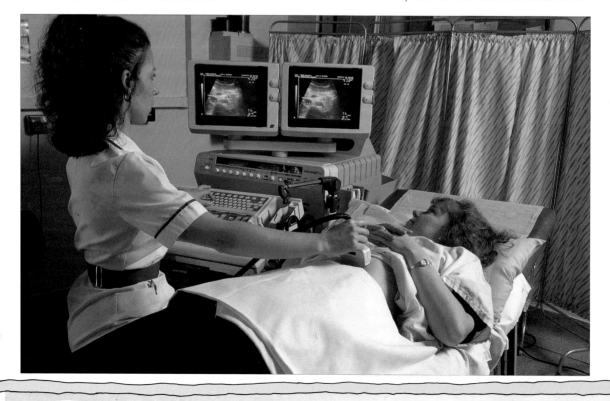

The heart pacemaker

Rune Elmqvist SWEDEN 1958

Electric signals in the heart keep it beating. They speed the beat up when you are exercising and slow it down when you are asleep. If this electrical system goes wrong and the heart beats too slowly, it can stop altogether. Artificial pacemakers deliver regular electric shocks to the heart to keep it beating.

The first pacemakers had batteries outside the body with a wire from them through a vein to the heart. They were all right for a short stay in hospital, but not for longer periods. Then, in 1958, Rune Elmqvist built a pacemaker to go inside the body. The mercury-zinc batteries were implanted under the skin. In 1960, Swedish doctor Ake Senning implanted one in a patient. The batteries lasted for two to three years before they had to be replaced.

In the 1980s, microprocessors were added so that the pacemaker was only triggered when the microprocessor detected that it was needed.

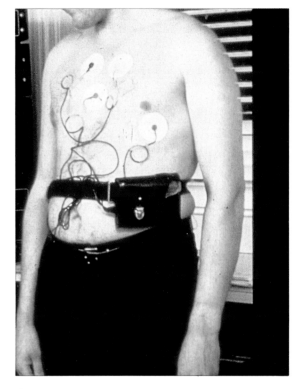

▲ This man is wearing a tracer which can provide twenty-four-hour monitoring for his heart.

Today's pacemakers are even more sophisticated. They regulate the heart according to the temperature of the blood. In 1988, a man was fitted with a nuclear pacemaker which uses a tiny piece of plutonium which should last for twenty years.

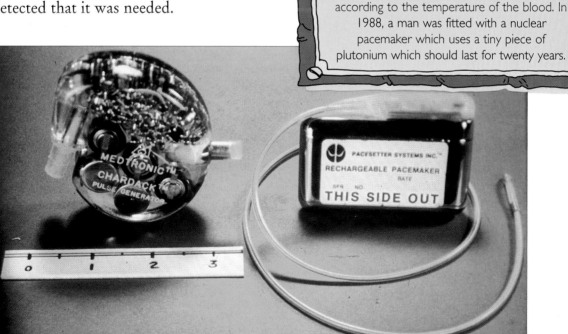

The link between smoking and death

Cuyler Hammond and Daniel Horn

UNITED STATES 1958

In 1958, Cuyler Hammond and Daniel Horn published the results of a startling and far-reaching study. For the first time, they showed that cigarette smoking not only causes lung cancer but also heart disease and many other fatal conditions.

Nearly twenty years earlier, a German doctor, F. H. Muller, had suggested that smoking causes lung cancer, a disease that, since World War I, had increased dramatically. In 1951, an American study had shown that out of 650 men who had lung cancer, over 620 of them had smoked cigarettes for over twenty-five years. In Britain, Richard Doll and Austin Hill had shown that, among 40,000 doctors, those that smoked heavily were ten times more likely to die of lung cancer than non-smokers. In the next ten years, the number of doctors who smoked halved.

Hammond and Horn, however, studied a larger number of men, nearly 200,000, for four years. Every time one of the men died, they found out whether the cause of death was linked to smoking. Almost half of the cigarette smokers who died, not just from lung cancer but from other diseases too, were killed by cigarette smoking.

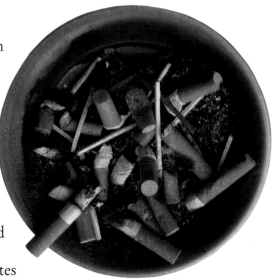

▼ A man's lungs drawn as ashtrays. His lungs are affected by each cigarette he smokes, however, once a person starts to smoke it is very difficult for them to give up.

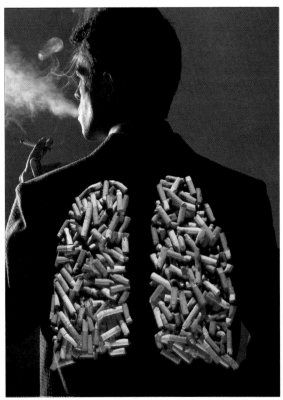

Cigarette companies make vast sums of money from making and selling cigarettes. After Hammond and Horn published their study, doctors and other people wanted their governments to ban cigarette advertising. They found, however, that governments will not impose a total ban because they do not want to lose the tax they collect from cigarette smokers.

Closed chest cardiac massage

W. B. Kouwenhoven UNITED STATES 1959

In 1926, the Consolidated Electric
Company of New York contacted the
Rockefeller Institute because they were
worried about the number of people who
were injured or killed by electric shocks. In
1928, Kouwenhoven began to investigate
ways of restarting a heart which has
stopped beating or is not beating properly.
Massaging the heart itself was one way, but
that involved opening up the chest in a
major operation. Another way was to pass
an electric current across the heart. Then Kouwenhoven
noticed that when the electricity was passed across the
heart, the chest reacted as though it had been thumped.
He wondered whether the heart could be started by
applying regular and rhythmic pressure from outside the
chest. He tried it on a cat whose heart had stopped
beating and it worked. Kouwenhoven experimented on
other animals and tried his method in hospitals.

In 1958, Henry Bahnson used
Kouwenhoven's technique to save the
life of a 2-year-old child. Since then
the method has been used by
doctors, ambulance men,
first aid workers
and others to
save the
lives of
thousands
of people.

One of the advantages of closed-chest
cardiac massage is that it can be given at the
site of an accident. If the heart stops beating
for more than a few minutes the blood is
starved of oxygen and can cause brain
damage. You can learn how to give this sort
of help in special first aid classes

▼ Paramedics try to restart
this person's heart and
breathing after he has fallen in
an accident. It is vital that they
get his heart beating before his
brain gets starved of oxygen.

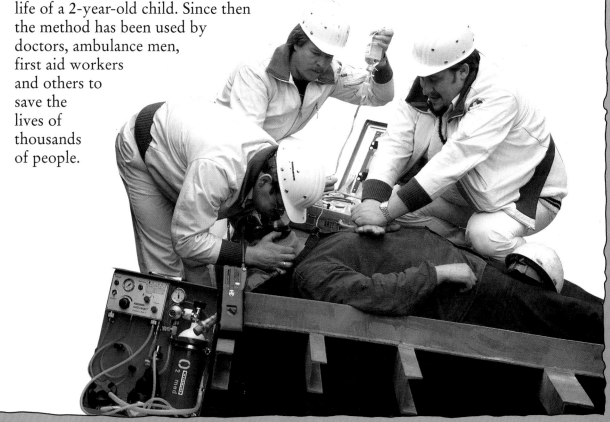

AVOIDING THE NEEDLE

Oral vaccination

Albert Sabin UNITED STATES 1961

There were two main problems with Salk's polio vaccine (see page 89). It was not completely effective against one of the three strains of polio and it only gave immunity for a limited time. Children had to be revaccinated regularly. Even as Salk's vaccination was being tested on thousands of children, Albert Sabin at the University of Cincinnati thought that he could produce a better one.

Salk's vaccine used samples of the virus which had been killed by formalin, but Sabin made a vaccine which used a small amount of live virus. He hoped it would give permanent immunity. Better still, it could be taken by mouth instead of being injected with a hypodermic needle. Between 1957 and 1959, Sabin tested his live virus in Mexico, Europe, Singapore and his native country, Russia. The trials were successful but the vaccine was not tried in the United States until 1961. In 1962, his vaccine became available and is now usually given instead of Salk's vaccine.

Franklin D. Roosevelt, president of the United States from 1933 to 1945, had been paralysed by polio. He was very keen to see the development of a vaccine against polio and encouraged the mass trials of the Salk vaccine in America. The authorities were so keen on the Salk vaccine they were slow to see the benefits of Sabin's.

▼ A nurse gives the polio vaccination to a child in India. The vaccine can also be given on a sugar cube.

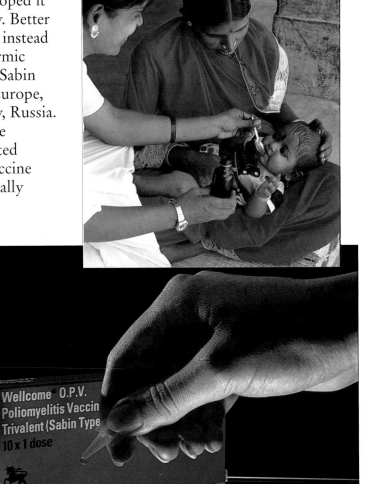

▶ The oral polio vaccine is given in three separate doses with intervals of one month between each dose. Reinforcing doses are given at school entry and school leaving.

Wellcome O.P.V.
Poliomyelitis Vaccin
Trivalent (Sabin Type
10 x 1 dose

Wellcome

Laser surgery

H. Vernon Ingram UNITED STATES 1964

In 1960, the American physicist T. H. Maiman built the first laser machine. Laser stands for 'Light Amplification by Stimulated Emission of Radiation'. The machine produces a very strong beam of radiation which can be aimed with absolute accuracy. Only four years later, H. Vernon Ingram used a laser in an eye operation.

Lasers are particularly successful in treating detached retinas. The retina at the back of the eyeball is packed with nerve endings which react to light by sending nerve signals to the brain. Sometimes, a small hole develops in the retina and fluid from inside the eye seeps through it. If the hole is not sealed, the retina will eventually become detached and the patient will go blind. However, it only takes a single pulse of laser light lasting just 0.001 seconds to weld the hole and prevent further damage.

In 1967, the Bell Telephone Company developed a laser which can cut and seal blood vessels at the same time. Lasers have made it possible to do many operations more quickly and with less scarring.

▶ A surgeon uses a hand-held laser instead of the traditional scalpel. Lasers are particularly useful for repairing the retina at the back of the eye and for making cuts without causing any bleeding. Haemophiliacs are people who cannot stop bleeding once they are cut, so this technique is very useful for treating them.

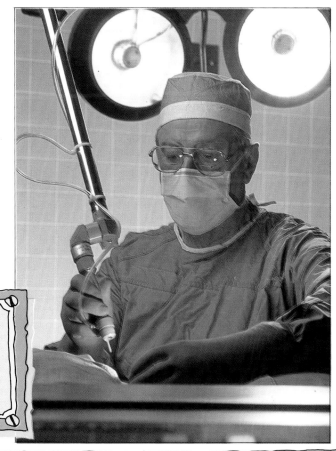

Lasers are used to treat cataracts and can be used with endoscopes and in microsurgery. A modern version of acupuncture uses a small laser beam instead of needles to avoid the risk of spreading the HIV virus.

Beta blockers

James Black UNITED KINGDOM 1964

In 1948, an American pharmacologist suggested that muscles have two kinds of receptors (which he called alpha and beta) which control the way the muscles, especially the heart, react to hormones such as adrenalin. Black realized that, if he could block the beta receptors, the heart would not have to work so hard when it was stimulated by a hormone. He discovered that the drug propranolol did just this.

Propranolol and other 'beta blockers' were quickly used to treat high blood pressure and other physical symptoms of stress, such as angina. Drug companies were very excited about them. They gave them to ski jumpers and racing drivers and filmed them in action to show that the beta blockers did not spoil their performance.

By 1974, however, doctors began to notice damaging side effects from beta blockers. Some patients developed heart failure and asthma was aggravated. However, newer and better beta blockers have been produced and these drugs are used extensively by doctors for treating heart problems.

In 1972, James Black also discovered another 'blocker', one which helped in the treatment of stomach ulcers. He found that the drug climetidine blocked the histamine receptors in the gut where ulcers tend to form.

▼ Scientists looked at the way athletes performed after they had been given beta blockers. Although it seemd to improve their performance, it was discovered that the drugs had side effects.

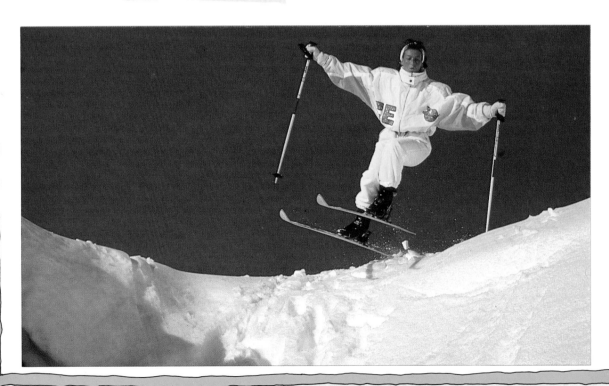

The endoscope
Harold Hopkins
UNITED KINGDOM 1965

An endoscope is a tube with a light which can be pushed through the mouth and down into the stomach, or through any other natural opening into the body. It is particularly useful to doctors because it allows them to see parts of the body that X-rays do not show. Using an endoscope a doctor can, for example, look at ulcers or tumours inside the stomach and so work out the best treatment for them.

The first endoscopes had a rigid tube and were invented over a hundred years ago. They were improved slowly but were not greatly used. Then, in the 1950s, endoscopes were made with flexible tubes so they could easily bend around corners inside the body, and in 1965, Harold Hopkins introduced rod lenses that gave a much clearer view. Today, endoscopes often have two glass-fibre tubes. The light is shone down one tube while the surgeon looks down the other or watches through a camera. Some endoscopes even have tiny microchip sensors which feed back information to a computer.

Some operations can be done using an endoscope and a laser. The endoscope includes an optical fibre which carries a laser beam for burning off growths and tumours and sealing burst blood vessels.

▲ Looking down an endoscope into the human stomach. An endoscope tube can be inserted into any natural opening, or through a small cut.

▼ An early endoscope, built in 1870, using a rigid tube instead of a rubber one.

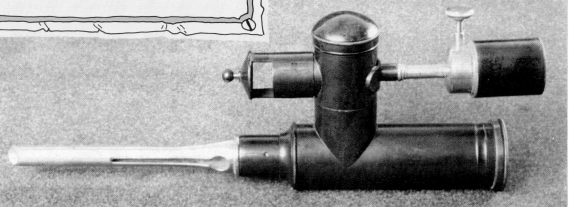

Artificial blood

Clark and Gollan UNITED STATES 1966

Clark and Gollan discovered that fluorocarbon, like blood, absorbs oxygen from the air. In 1966, these two researchers dropped some mice into a tank of liquid and held them below the surface. The mice should have drowned within minutes, but instead they stayed alive for a few hours. The liquid in the tank contained fluorocarbon and water. The molecules of fluorocarbon linked with some of the oxygen in the water and passed into the mice's blood. Clark and Gollan had taken the first step towards inventing a substitute for blood.

The next year another American, Henry Sloviter, injected some rabbits with a mixture which contained fluorocarbon and egg white. He found that the rabbits could survive provided the mixture did not replace more than a third of their blood.

The first human to receive artificial blood was the Japanese researcher Ryochi Naito. In 1979, he injected himself with 200 ml (nearly half a pint) of the milky fluid. Now doctors have several different formulas for artificial blood for use in emergencies.

▼ This artificial blood contains man-made haemoglobin. Haemoglobin is the oxygen-carrying molecule in the blood, and looks red in colour when it is carrying a lot of oxygen.

Artificial blood is only used along with human blood in a blood transfusion. It is often given to patients who need large amount of blood, such as those who are suffering from third degree burns.

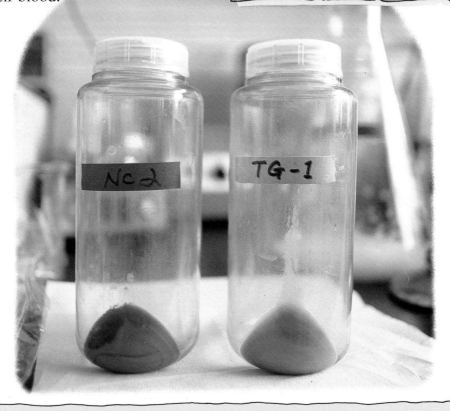

THREE-DIMENSIONAL PICTURES

CAT scans

G. N. Hounsfield UNITED KINGDOM 1967

G. N. Hounsfield was an electrical engineer and computer expert who decided to see if computers could be used to improve the quality of X-ray photographs. He developed a CAT scanner which gives a three-dimensional picture of 'slices' or sections through the body.

CAT stands for 'Computerized Axial Tomography'. A CAT scanner feeds narrow beams of X-rays through the patient's body. The X-ray detector rotates around the patient, and records the density of different kinds of tissues. In this way, pictures of the brain, of organs or of whole sections of the body can be made. Later CAT scanners could shade the different densities of tissue in different colours, giving even clearer pictures.

CAT scans allow surgeons to get a good look at diseased organs before they operate. They also help them to diagnose illnesses.

> NMR machines also give 3D pictures of the body. Instead of using X-rays, which can be harmful, they use magnetism to make hydrogen inside the body resonate or vibrate. NMR machines can examine atoms and molecules and are particularly useful with organ transplants. NMR stands for 'Nuclear Magnetic Resonance'.

▼ A CAT scan of the lungs shown in blue/green.

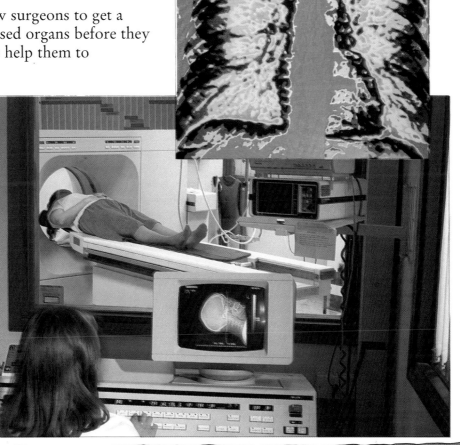

101

Heart transplants
Christiaan Barnard SOUTH AFRICA 1967

In 1967, newspapers and television broke the amazing news that Dr Christiaan Barnard had transplanted a heart from one person to another. There had been many less successful attempts.

In 1961, Norman Shumway transplanted a heart from one dog to another. The new heart worked for three weeks before the dog's body rejected it. Three years later, a patient in Mississippi was given a chimpanzee's heart, but it was not large enough to cope and soon failed. In 1967, Christiaan Barnard took the heart of a 24-year-old woman who was dying of head injuries and transplanted it into the body of Louis Washkansky, a 54-year-old man who was dying of heart disease. Washkansky lived for eighteen days before he died of pneumonia. Twenty years later, hospitals were carrying out heart transplants on patients who often lived for five years or more following their operation.

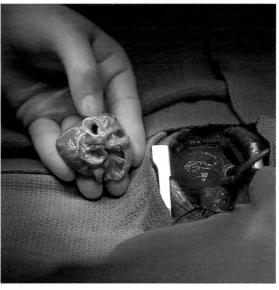

▲ On the left is the tiny heart which needed replacing. On the right, now in position, is the new, normal-sized heart. This operation was performed on a 2-month-old baby.

One of the biggest problems in transplanting organs from one person to another is overcoming the patient's immune system. The natural reaction of the body is to reject the incoming organ, even when blood groups and tissues have been matched as closely as possible. Drugs are used to suppress this immune response.

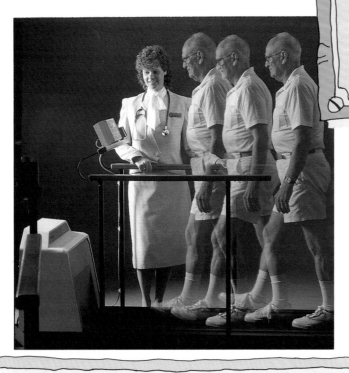

◀ A heart transplant patient has his progress checked carefully by the nurse using this monitoring machine. Transplants are limited by a shortage of organ donors and a lack of money. In India, people sell their kidneys to doctors, but in this country it is considered 'unethical'.

Microsurgery
Komatsu and Tamai
UNITED STATES 1968

Perhaps some of the most amazing feats in surgery have been the successful rejoining of fingers, hands, arms and feet which have been cut off in accidents with machinery or in motor crashes. To rejoin a limb and get it to work again, blood vessels and nerves as well as skin and bone have to be sewn together.

The way was opened as long ago as 1912, when Alexis Carrell invented a way of sewing larger blood vessels together. In the 1960s, better microscopes, fine needles and fine silk threads made it possible to sew together even small blood vessels. But the last step, rebuilding shattered nerves, only became possible in 1967. In 1968, Komatsu and Tamai used all these new techniques when they rejoined a severed thumb.

One problem in rejoining severed limbs is that the smallest blood vessels do not open at once. Blood is pumped into the limb but it cannot get out again. The problem can be solved by applying leeches to remove the excess blood.

> Leeches were once used to treat all kinds of illness. They were attached to the flesh and allowed to suck up to twenty-five grams (half an ounce) of blood. When they were removed, the blood continued to flow, because the leech injects a substance which stopped the blood from clotting.

▼ Two surgeons look down one microscope so that they both see exactly the same view of the operation. Microsurgery involves repairing fine tissue and making tiny stitches to sew nerves and blood vessels.

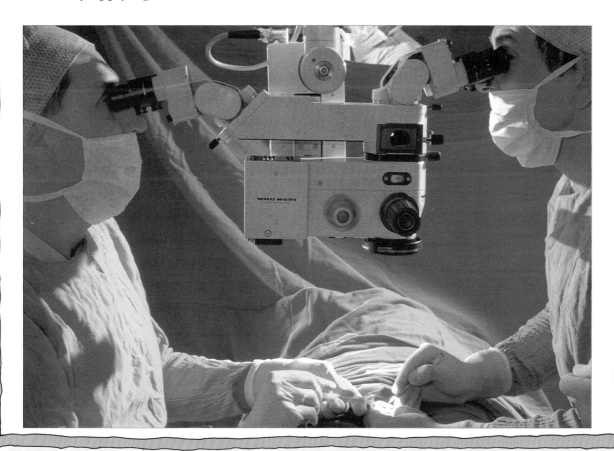

Artificial hearts

Robert Jarvik UNITED STATES 1970

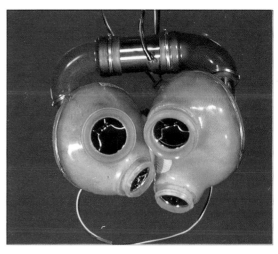

In 1957, Willem Kolff, who had earlier made the first artificial kidney for humans (see page 84), also made an artificial heart. He implanted it into a dog, but the dog died an hour and a half later. Then, in 1970, Robert Jarvik, working at the University of Utah, developed another artificial heart, which he called the 'Jarvik 7'. It was made of glass-fibre and polyurethane, and used compressed air to pump the blood through the body. Jarvik tested it on several young calves, but, since the heart could not grow as they grew, they all died after about sixty-six days.

▲ A Jarvik 7 heart which will pump the blood around the body in place of the orginal, diseased heart. In an average lifetime, the heart will beat three billion times.

In 1982, a Jarvik heart was implanted into a person for the first time. Barney Clarke was 61 years old, and lived for 112 days with his new heart. This success encouraged other surgeons around the world. About ninety people received Jarvik hearts, and William Schroeder lived for twenty months, longer than any of the others. However, people were shocked when they saw on television how much Schroeder suffered, and artificial hearts were then banned in the United States.

Since artificial hearts were banned, scientists have developed other devices to help the heart do its work. In 1989, Richard Wampler made a tiny turbine called a 'Hemopump' which can take over from the heart for a short time, and, in 1990, an American company developed a heart assistance device which can be implanted in the body.

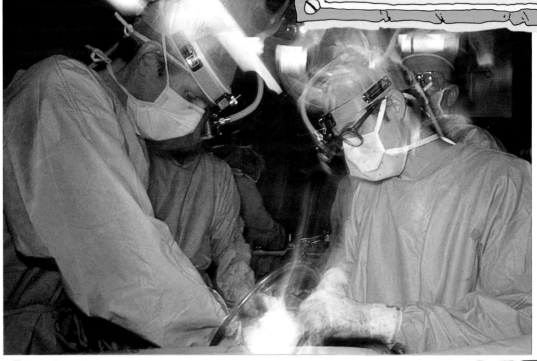

In vitro fertilization

Patrick Steptoe UNITED KINGDOM 1978

For conception to take place, an egg cell travels from the woman's ovary down her Fallopian tube into the womb. It is here that the egg meets a barrage of sperm, one of which must successfully penetrate it for a new life to begin. If a woman's Fallopian tubes are blocked, conception cannot occur. In 1969, Patrick Steptoe and Robert Edwards removed some eggs from a patient's ovaries and fertilized them with her husband's sperm. It took nearly ten years' more work before Steptoe achieved his aim. He kept the eggs and sperm on a glass dish for several days to make sure that conception had taken place. Then the fertilized egg was put back into the mother's uterus (womb) and left to develop normally. In 1978, Louise Brown, the first baby to be fertilized outside the womb, was born. Since then many other couples have given birth using Steptoe's methods.

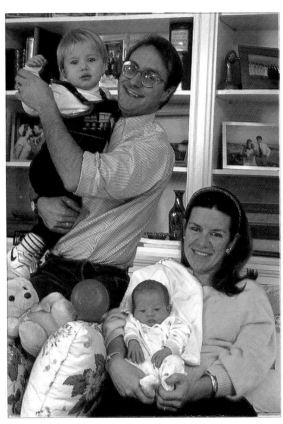

In vitro fertilization, or 'IVF', is used to help many kinds of infertility. If the husband cannot produce sperm, sperm from a sperm bank may be used instead. Several fertilized eggs are usually replaced in the mother's womb because the chances of success are still very low.

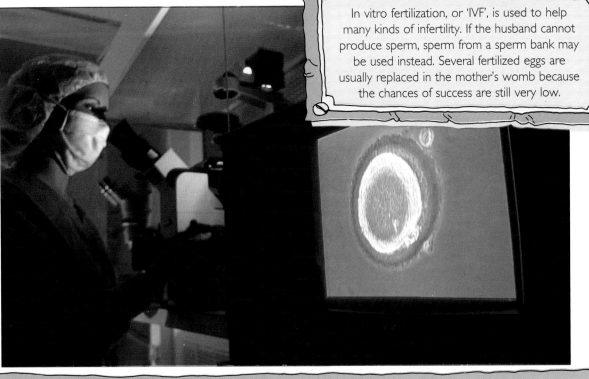

Artificial skin

Ioannis Yannis UNITED STATES 1981

Your skin not only keeps dirt and germs out, it also stops moisture escaping from inside your body. When a large area of skin is badly burnt or damaged, doctors have to act quickly to replace the fluid and protect the wound. If only the top layers of skin are damaged new skin will grow, but when a patient suffers very serious burns the skin cannot repair itself. Usually a thin layer of skin is taken from another part of the body and grafted over the wound.

Artificial skin is used to provide a basis for the graft. It is made from a polymer (a long, chain-like molecule) combined with other chemicals, including a substance extracted from shark's cartilage. Ioannis Yannas was the first person to use artificial skin to treat a third-degree burn. Today, it is used in the first stage of a skin graft. The artificial skin protects the wound from infection and encourages connective tissue to grow. The body's immune system gradually breaks down the polymer, but when a layer of the patient's own skin is grafted over the top of it, it heals quickly.

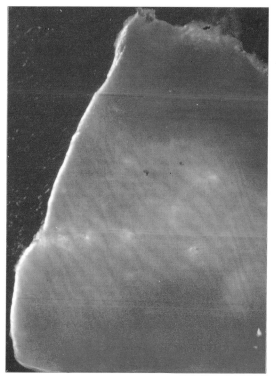

▲ Synthetic skin is made by starting with a piece of real skin and 'growing' some more from it. Skin is one of the major organs of the body. It can totally renew itself within about sixty days.

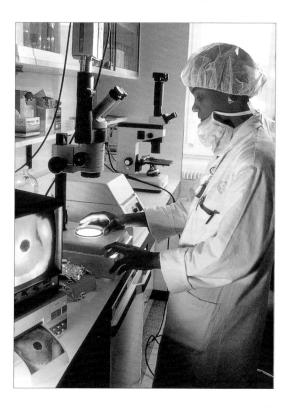

In the 1980s, Anthony Sun experimented with an artificial pancreas which contained beta cells. Insulin is made by beta cells. His work may one day lead to the development of a new cure for diabetes (see page 74).

▲ Artificial skin displayed on a monitor. Artificial skin today is easily accepted by the human body, and can even be frozen for use in the future.

IDENTIFYING THE CAUSE OF AIDS

Human immuno-deficiency virus

Luc Montagnier FRANCE 1984

In 1981, health officials in the United States noticed that more and more people were dying from very rare diseases or diseases that did not usually kill. At first, all the victims seemed to be homosexual men, but, within a few months, they were joined by drug addicts and men and women who had received blood transfusions. Each was dying because their own immune system was no longer working. Doctors called the new disease 'Acquired Immuno-Deficiency Syndrome', or AIDS.

Scientists suspected that the disease was caused by a virus and, in 1984, a team in France led by Luc Montagnier isolated and identified the virus which attacked and destroyed white blood cells (see page 55). The virus was called the Human Immuno-deficiency Virus (HIV). It can be passed from one person to another in blood, or through having sex, and it may be several years before the person actually develops AIDS.

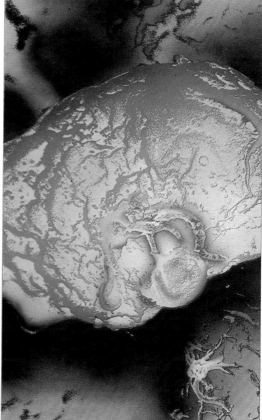

▲ View down an electron microscope of the AIDS virus (orange) budding from a white blood cell. White blood cells form the basis of the human immune system which is almost completely broken down by AIDS.

At the moment there is no cure for AIDS, but people are encouraged to avoid the disease by taking preventive measures, such as practising 'safe sex' by using condoms, and not sharing syringe needles. Donated blood is treated to make sure there is no HIV virus present.

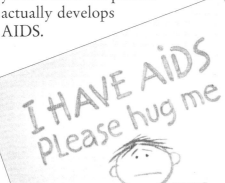

◀ You cannot catch AIDS from touching a person who has it. It is very important that we learn as much as possible about this disease and pass that information on to people living all over the world so that we can stop it spreading further. It is only through creating greater awareness that the progress of this disease can be slowed.

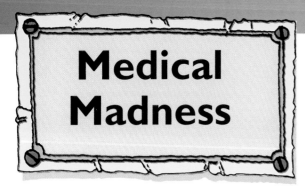

Medical Madness

Solve each clue and fill in the missing letters in the word next to it. The words in **bold** type in the clues tell you which item in the book contains the answer.

When you have filled in all the spaces, the first letters of each of the words read downwards to make two other words – for which your clue is: A promise that doctors make in *Caring for the Patient.*

The letters 1-15 taken in order make another word that describes how medical discoveries are often made.

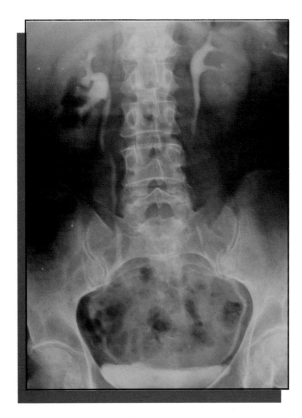

_E_ A _ _ _ (1) — Their activity was first measured by William Einthoven's **Electrocardiograph**

I _ _ _ I _ _E_ (4) — An **Ophthalmoscope** can see this part of the eye

_ O _I_ O _ (13) — **Antibodies** can destroy this kind of substance in the body

_ _ A _ U E (3) — An illness carried by rats, or any widespread disease, as studied in **The Science of Epidemiology**

O_ _ _ _ E _ (14) — In **Respiration** this is absorbed into the blood

_ O _ _ O _ (2) — The illness for which Edward Jenner originally developed an antidote, later known as **Smallpox Vaccine**

_ U _ E _ (5) — Gloves worn for **Safer Surgery**

A _ _ I _ A (15) — Pain in the chest sometimes treated by **Beta Blockers**

_ _ I A _ _ (10) — Tests to determine the safety and effectiveness of the **Polio Vaccine**

I_ _ E _ _ (6) — You could do this with a **Hypodermic Syringe**

_ O _ A _ (12) — A metal used to treat cancer in **Radiotherapy**

O _ _ A _ _ (11) — In the body, in **Heart Transplants**, they work; outside the body, they play!

A _ _ _ U _ (7) — A place where mental patients used to be kept until the discovery of **Hypnosis**

_ _ E _ E (8) — The fly that carries **Sleeping Sickness**

_ A _ _ E _ (9) — He discovered that **Leprosy** was caused by a germ

Answers can be found on page 111 at the back of the book

Index

Picture Acknowledgements

The publishers would also like to thank:
Glasgow University Library; Prado, Madrid; Royal College of Surgeons, London; Royal Society, London; Museum of the History of Science, Oxford; Eton College, Windsor.

a = above, b = below

Art Directors Photo Library: 91b;
Biophoto Associates: 10b; 21a; 24a; 30b; 39b; 43a; 49b; 51a; 53a; 59a; 63a; 64b; 73b; 87a.
Bridgeman Art Library: 13b (Eton College Windsor); 16b (Glasgow University Library); 22b (Museum of the History of Science, Oxford); 28a (Royal College of Surgeons, London); 69a (Royal Society, London); 73a (Prado, Madrid).
E.T. Archive: 8a; 14b; 19a; 41a; 46a; 61b; 68b; 76b.
Mary Evans Picture Library: 8b; 11b; 12; 13a; 16a; 17a; 21b; 27a; 31b; 32b; 34a; 38a; 40b; 43b; 44a; 45b; 46b; 47a; 47b; 50b; 56a; 56b; 58a; 62; 64a; 67b; 76a. Format: 90b (Brenda Prince): 107b (Brenda Prince).
Sally and Richard Greenhill: 29a; 33a; 36a; 85a; 86a.
Robert Harding Picture Library: 9 (Rainbird); 20 (Rainbird); 25b (Images); 29b (Orbis); 33b (Rainbird); 34b (Lorraine Wilson); 36b (DK Holdsworth); 40a (Walter Rawlings); 44b (M. Leslie Evans); 45a (Paolo Koch); 51b (John Stathatos); 52 (Rainbird); 53b; 57b (J.E. Stevenson); 61a (Orbis); 65a (Joe Clarke); 65b (Peter Blackwell); 66b (Bildagentur Schuster); 69b (Bildagentur Schuster / Stone); 80a (J.E Stevenson); 83a (Rainbird); 84b (Explorer /M. Cambazard); 90a (Orbis); 92 (M. Leslie Evans); 93b (Photri); 94a (IMS AB); 95 (Bildagentur Schuster / Schiller); 98 (Explorers/C. Thorens); 101b (M. Leslie Evans). Images Colour: 50a.
The Hulton-Deutsch Collection: 60b.
Science Photo Library: 11a; 15b; 18b; 22a; 23; 24b; 26b; 31a; 37a; 38b; 39a; 41b; 48a; 54a; 54b; 55b; 57a; 58b; 59b; 60a; 63b; 66a; 67a; 68a; 71a; 71b; 72b; 74; 75a; 77a; 77b; 78; 79; 80b; 81a; 81b; 82a; 82b; 83b; 84a; 85b; 86b; 87b; 88; 89a; 89b; 91a; 94b; 96a; 96b; 97a; 97b; 99a; 100; 101a; 102a; 102b; 103; 104a; 104b; 105a; 105b; 106a; 106b; 107a.

Wellcome Institute Library, London: 10a; 14a; 15a; 17b; 18a; 19b; 20a; 25a; 26a; 27b; 28b; 30a; 32a (National Medical Slide Bank); 35a; 35b; 37b; 42; 48b (National Medical Slide Bank); 49a; 55a; 70; 72a; 75b (National Medical Slide Bank); 93a (National Medical Slide Bank); 99b.

Front cover (clockwise from top left): Biophoto Associates; Biophoto Associates; Science Photo Library; Science Photo Library; Science Photo Library; Biophoto Associates; Science Photo Library; Science Photo Library; Science Photo Library; Science Photo Library; Science Photo Library; Science Photo Library.

Back cover (clockwise from top left): Mary Evans Picture Library; Robert Harding Picture Library (Bildagentur Schuster / Stone); Science Photo Library; Mary Evans Picture Library; Wellcome Institute Library, London; Science Photo Library; Biophoto Associates; Robert Harding Picture Library (M. Leslie Evans); Robert Harding Picture Library (M. Leslie Evans); Wellcome Institute Library, London.

Introduction
Mary Evans Picture Library: 3a (left); 3b. Robert Harding Picture Library: 3a (IMS.AB) (right); 4b (Bildagentur Schuster /Schiller; 4b (J.E. Stevenson). Wellcome Institute Library, London: 4a.

Puzzle (clockwise from top left)
Wellcome Institute Library, London Wellcome Institute Library, London Wellcome Institute Library, London, E.T. Archive, Science Photo Library, Wellcome Institute Library, London, Wellcome Institute Library, London Mary Evans Picture Library, Mary Evans Picture Library, Wellcome Institute Library, London.